From the editors of
Health

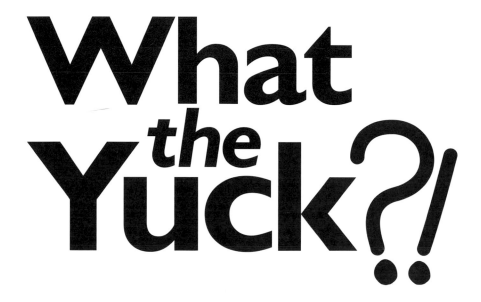

ISBN-13: 978-0-8487-3417-6
ISBN-10: 0-8487-3417-3
Library of Congress Control Number: 2009943612
Printed in the United States of America
First Printing 2010

Health

Editor in Chief: Ellen Kunes
Creative Director: Ben Margherita
Executive Editor: Lisa Lombardi
Managing Editor: Faustina S. Williams
West Coast Editor: Jen Furmaniak (JB Talent)
West Coast Associate: Rachel Goldman (JB Talent)
Deputy Editor: Jennifer Brunnemer Slaton
Beauty and Fashion Editor: Colleen Sullivan
Beauty and Fashion News Editor: Jennifer Goldstein
Senior Editor: Su Reid-St. John
Senior Food and Nutrition Editor: Frances A. Largeman-Roth, RD
Medical Editor: Roshini Rajapaksa, MD
Associate Editors: Shaun A. Chavis, Susan Hall
Assistant Editor: Rozalynn S. Frazier
Office Manager: Stephanie Wolford
Editorial Assistants: Leslie Barrie, Caylin Harris, Kimberly Holland, Melanie Rud
Editorial Interns: Diana Cerqueira, Ashley Macha

ART DEPARTMENT
Design Director: José Fernandez
Senior Designer: Amanda Stevens

PHOTO DEPARTMENT
Photo Director: Marybeth Welsh Dulany
Contributing Photo Editors: Inna Khavinson, Vanessa Griggs
Art Production Assistant: Jamie Blair

COPY AND RESEARCH
Copy Chief: Tanya M. Hines-Wright
Research Editor: Michael Gollust
Assistant Copy Editor: Shannon Friedmann Hatch

PRODUCTION
Production Coordinator: Lauren A. Wade

HEALTH.COM
Editorial Director: Ellen Kunes
Editor in Chief: Amy O'Connor
Executive Editor: Theresa Tamkins
Associate Editor: Ray Hainer
Assistant Editors: Mara Betsch, Kate Stinchfield

From the editors of
Health

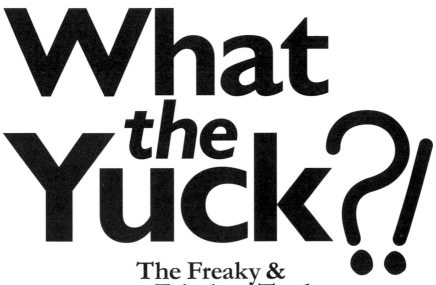

What
the
Yuck?!

The Freaky &
Fabulous Truth
About Your Body

BY ROSHINI RAJ, MD
with LISA LOMBARDI

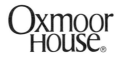

Oxmoor
House®

To my parents for their constant
devotion and for teaching me that
dreams should have no limits.
To my husband for his selfless
and unflagging support (and for
his midnight massages).
And to my sons, whose smiles
remind me daily of the infinite
possibilities of love.

—Roshini Rajapaksa, MD

ACKNOWLEDGMENTS

What the Yuck?! is a huge group effort and we are incredibly grateful for the contributions and cheerleading we received along the way. There would be no Yuck without Health Editor in Chief Ellen Kunes, who wasn't afraid to go there, so that we could answer the real stuff that keeps women up at night. She had the vision for a women's health guide that blended good information with good humor, and we're very thankful she championed this book.

Also, big thanks to the extra-creative Creative Director of Health, Ben Margherita, for his amazing design and illustrations (Ben, who knew you could draw?!). Health editorial assistant Kimberly Holland was this book's secret hero, spending hours and hours doing fast and smart reporting...and anything else needed.

A huge thank you to Sylvia Auton and John L. Brown, for being such wonderful champions of Health, and for giving us all the tools we needed to create this book. We're also immensely grateful to the team at Time Home Entertainment Inc. and Oxmoor House: Richard Fraiman, Jim Childs, Susan Payne Dobbs, Katherine Cobbs, Sydney Webber, Fonda Hitchcock, Emily Chappell, and Laurie Herr.

We couldn't have created the book you hold in your hands without the staffs of Health and Health.com, especially Dave Watt, Frances Largeman-Roth, RD, Leslie Barrie, Marybeth Welsh Dulany, José Fernandez, Michael Gollust, Jennifer Slaton, Amy O'Connor, and Theresa Tamkins. Thanks also to Anne Krueger for her work on the column, Helen Wan for advising us, and Debra Richman and Amanda Potters and their teams for helping us get the word out.

ROSHINI WOULD LIKE TO THANK:

Suzy Alvarez, Joy Bauer, Jim Bell, Shri Bhat, Edmund Bini, MD, Andrew Brotman, MD, Rachana Choubey, Jim Clinton, Ann Curry, Janet Flora, Kathie Lee Gifford, Michael Glantz, Lester Holt, Brian Jacobs, Edna de Jesus, Elene Kolb, Hoda Kotb, Matt Lauer, Lisa Lombardi, Laura Malick, Natalie Morales, Sucheta Nasta, Mehmet Oz, MD, Eve Pearl, Robert Raicht, MD, Amy Robach, Al Roker, Andrew Rubin, Yardena Schwartz, Marc Siegel, MD, Lindsay Sobel, Elizabeth Weinshel, MD, Meredith Vieira, Marc Victor, Gerald Villanueva, MD and Jenna Wolfe

LISA WOULD LIKE TO THANK:

Roshini Rajapaksa, MD for bringing not just her medical smarts but her imagination to this book.

My amazing husband, Dan Bova, and sons Henry and Gus for putting up with the late nights. You're truly the best.

My parents, for being my early and forever examples of the power of hard work.

My friends and co-workers for sharing questions: Your healthy curiosity (or shall we call it neurosis?) took this book to a more real place.

I'd also like to thank all the doctors who've fielded my embarrassing questions over the years. It takes a true professional to keep a straight face when a patient says: "I'm here because a dead mouse fell on my face."

CONTENTS

"Dr. Raj's willingness to take on any kind of body problem in a smart, reassuring, real way has made her *What the Yuck?!* column the most popular health page in our magazine."

—Ellen Kunes
Editor in Chief
Health Magazine

Dear Readers,

We all have them: those questions we think are just too embarrassing to ask our doctors. Whether they're minor worries ("What is that ugly white gunk on the bottom of my feet?") or truly terrifying health concerns ("Can my cell phone give me cancer?") we want answers that cut through the confusion and help us feel more in control.

For three years, Roshini Rajapaksa, MD—known here at *Health* and on the *TODAY* show as Dr. Raj—has been answering tough questions like these for women across America. Dr. Raj's willingness to take on any kind of body problem in a smart, reassuring, real way has made her **What the Yuck?!** column the most popular health page in our magazine.

So we had a great idea: Why not bring Dr. Raj's candid advice to even more women? Our goal was simple: to address every kind of question we all have—on sex, men's bodies, dating, pregnancy, Hollywood health fads—in one brilliant book. I think the result is something totally new and exciting: a completely frank and, yes, even fun women's health guide. What I love most is that Dr. Raj is willing to go there, weighing in on everything from cupcake headaches to the infection you can get from your skinny jeans.

To make it easier to find what you're looking for, we've organized **What the Yuck?!** by topic (from "In the Loo" and "Between the Sheets" to "On A Date" and "Life 3.0"). But it's also a blast to flip through and dip into. We hope you find this book reassuring, surprising, informative, entertaining, and incredibly useful. I know it will help you to feel great every single day.

Enjoy!

Ellen Kunes
Editor in Chief
Health magazine
Editorial Director
Health.com

INTRODUCTION

It happens every day. A woman walks into my office, blushing and avoiding eye contact. When I ask why she came to see me, she starts mumbling under her breath, and when I reassure her she can tell me anything, she finally blurts out, "I am so embarrassed to say this, but I have a lot of gas!"

Embarrassed? Please! I talk about gas, poop, and other exciting bodily functions several hours a day! And I spent precious years of my life studying and training just so I could talk about these topics. Once I explain to my stressed-out patient that there are absolutely no off-limit subjects, I can see the anxiety dissolve from her face. And then we can get down to the nitty-gritty, delve into what is really going on, and hopefully start to help.

I get it. It's not easy to discuss smelly discharge, nipple hairs, or any of the hundreds of topics our grandmothers taught us "nice ladies" don't discuss in public. But talking does help: We learn more about our bodies, which can make us feel so much better, both physically and emotionally.

And truth is, not talking can hurt us in very real ways. Ignoring a symptom because it's uncomfortable to bring up can be hazardous to your health.

That's why it was so important to me to write this book. I want you to know you're not alone (we all wonder about the same stuff) and no question is too weird or gross or random to bring up to a doctor. I've heard it all (as you can tell from the question on page 64, I'm pretty unshockable), I've been there too, and I am ready to help.

—Dr. Raj

In the Loo

chapter

1

Potty talk for grown-up girls

1: In the Loo

Q. *"Sometimes when I laugh or sneeze I leak pee—I thought that was just something old ladies did!"*

a Back away from the adult diapers—you are not there yet! I know lots of women with this problem, and while it can be embarrassing, it's not a sign you're skipping right to your golden years. What you most likely have is stress incontinence, which causes you to lose a little pee when you laugh, cough, sneeze, or do anything that puts pressure on your bladder. Weakening in the muscles that support your bladder and urethra is usually to blame. As a result, when the urges come, you might just lose a little control down there—or worse, a lot.

Limiting fluid intake—especially alcohol and caffeine, which tend to race through your system—will help. Pee as soon as you wake up and right before bed. And when you feel the urge to go, do so as soon as possible. That'll keep stress off those muscles and prevent stretching of your bladder walls.

Kegel exercises (yep, the same ones that make sex feel better) can help by strengthening the muscles. While sitting in your chair, imagine you're holding in urine. Hold for 10 seconds and relax for 10 seconds; repeat 10 to 15 times, three times a day. As you build up these muscles (over the course of several weeks) the leakage should let up. (If it doesn't stop in a month or so, visit your doctor.) In the meantime, you can avoid an embarrassing leak by throwing on a panty liner before you go out.

Q. I always feel like I have a urinary tract infection—I have a dragging down pain in my abdomen, and I have to pee constantly without much coming out. But every time I get tested, the doctor says I'm fine. Is it all just in my head?

Don't worry, you're not crazy. It sounds like you have painful bladder syndrome (or interstitial cystitis), a real and frustrating condition in which chronic inflammation of your bladder brings on frequent, and sometimes very sudden and painful, urges to urinate. It can even cause incontinence (see the Q & A at left).

A urologist can diagnose you and offer solutions that work. Among them: Cut back on caffeine and alcohol, both of which send you dashing to the ladies' room. You'll also want to stay at a healthy weight because extra pounds put pressure on, and can even weaken, your pelvic floor muscles. Your urologist may also prescribe antispasmodic medications—they relax your bladder's muscles and thus prevent the contractions that lead to frequency and urgency.

The latest treatment? Injecting Botox into the bladder muscles. This isn't to give you a younger-looking urinary tract but rather to paralyze the overactive muscles. But the paralysis is only temporary, so this isn't considered a great option for long-term relief. As a last resort, there's surgery—but thankfully, most women find relief without having to hit the operating room.

· · · · · · ·

Q. Why is my pee so dark after running?

Sounds like you're dehydrated. When we lose a lot of fluid (as we do through heavy sweating when we're running or exercising), our body reacts by concentrating the urine and absorbing as much usable water as it can to maintain the right balance of fluids. So essentially, it's just making your pee more potent—hence, the darker color.

48 ounces
That's how much we pee each day.

Before you even lace up your running shoes, drink up (16-20 ounces 2 hours before, and 4-8 ounces 10 minutes before you exercise). Also sip fluids during your run and after it, too. Try to avoid alcohol and caffeine on days you'll be doing long runs as they can make you even more dehydrated.

• • • • • • •

Q. Can I pass my UTI to my guy during sex? How would he know he has it?

In terms of run-of-the-mill urinary tract infections (UTIs) caused by bacteria, no, they're not contagious. These UTIs can't be passed person-to-person, so no need to worry about passing yours on. That means you can't get one from him either. (If you or he has an uncommon UTI caused by yeast or an STD like *Trichomonas vaginalis*, then it *can* be passed back and forth though.) You generally catch a UTI from yourself when the bacteria in your rectum and anus get into your vagina and travel up into your urinary tract, setting up shop. But sex may make your UTI worse, so it's best to lay off the bedroom action until you've been on an antibiotic for 24 hours.

• • • • • • •

Q. The more sex I have, the more UTIs I get! What can I do—short of taking a vow of celibacy?

You poor thing. Unfortunately, some of us are just more prone to these annoying infections. In fact, 80 percent of women who have had at least two infections will have recurrences. The good news: You can have a healthy sex life *and* a healthy urinary tract. Just follow these three simple rules:

SIMPLE RULE #1 FOR PREVENTING UTIS:
Drink plenty of water and cranberry juice. Water really does flush out your system. And drinking cranberry juice isn't just

67%
of women have been too embarrassed about a health concern to bring it up to their doc.
Source: Health.com poll

an old wives' tale—it's a natural way to speed up recovery from and prevent future urinary tract infections. Two 4-ounce glasses a day of the red stuff is ideal.

SIMPLE RULE #2 FOR PREVENTING UTIS:
Wear cotton underwear. Cotton has a key advantage over silk and polyester: It's breathable, so you sweat less in it, leaving less dampness for bacteria to flourish.

SIMPLE RULE #3 FOR PREVENTING UTIS:
Empty your bladder before and after sex. And, if you're especially prone to UTIs, wash your vagina before and after as well. Why bother? This eliminates bacteria before it has a chance to transfer to your urethra and work its way inside and up the tract.

· · · · · · ·

Q. Which sex positions are most likely to give me a urinary tract infection?

There really isn't one move that is a disaster for your bladder, though there are some that are worse than others. Any position that irritates the urethra (like woman on top or the man riding high on the woman's pelvis) can lead to UTIs. Another pesky one: rear entry. When the man goes from anal sex to vaginal sex, he's transferring fecal bacteria. That bacteria works its way up the urinary tract, and in a few days—hello, infection.

· · · · · · ·

Q. This is embarrassing, but lately my bowel movements are green. What could that mean?

Okay, deep breath. If you see something out of the ordinary (i.e., not in the brown palette), you can usually chalk it up to food. After all, what goes in must come out. Leafy greens (which contain chlorophyll and can turn stool

HOW **BAD** IS IT *REALLY?*

To take laxatives to lose a couple of pounds quick.

To be honest, it's not terrible—but you won't accomplish much. Here's why: You're only losing the weight of the poop you flush out. As soon as you eat again, more stool will form, and your weight will go right back to where it was. (And while laxatives aren't physically addictive, some dieters get psychologically hooked and pop them frequently, which can be harmful.) My suggestion? Skip it.

green) or even artificial food coloring (in everything from that vivid-green pistachio ice cream to St. Patrick's Day cupcakes) can alter the hue of your poo, as can medicines and supplements.

It's normal for our stool to be green higher up in our digestive tract where green bile mixes with digested food. But it gets darker as it moves farther down. So if you're still seeing green at the other end, it might mean things are moving through your system really fast. This is probably just the result of something you ate or drank—caffeine or acidic foods (like citrus juices) are notorious for sending us racing to the rest room. And certain allergies and intolerances (super-spicy curry comes to mind) also put things on the fast track.

Most diet-related stool-color changes will clear up in a day or two after the food makes its way through your system. But if the unusual color persists or changes to red or even black; or if you have other symptoms like constant urges to go to the bathroom, vomiting, or stomach cramps, do see your doctor promptly.

● ● ● ● ● ●

Q. How bad is it to sit on a public toilet seat? Could I catch something nasty?

It's not as bad as you think. There are actually more germs on the floor in a public bathroom (hang up your purse!) than on the toilet seat. If the bathroom seems especially gross, use a paper cover if available, or just cover the seat with toilet paper.

But don't worry too much about contracting a sexually transmitted disease from your rest room pit stops. The fact is, if you have a healthy immune system, you'll be able to resist whatever germs you're exposed to while on the john. If you're really worried about germs, look for stalls that have covers over most of the toilet paper roll. When a toilet is flushed it sprays germs and microscopic fecal matter into the air (lovely, I know). But if the toilet paper is protected, you're far less likely to spread germs on yourself as you wipe.

Why does my doctor need to know *that?*

You think your MD is just being nosy when she asks about
your sex life or how many drinks you knock back. But
I promise, there is a good reason for us to go there.

 SEXUAL HISTORY: What's it to us? Doctors screen for cervical
cancer and other diseases based on sexual history. And we need to know
whether you could have been exposed to sexually transmitted diseases
(STDs) because they often present with subtle symptoms.

 EXACTLY WHAT YOU DO IN BED: I know asking about anal
intercourse seems *way* too personal. But if you come in complaining of
rectal pain or bleeding, this info will help your doc understand the likely
culprit. Also, there are certain diseases—such as HPV and gonorrhea—
that are more commonly transmitted through the "back door."

IF YOU EVER LIT UP (AND WHEN): Even smoking just one
cigarette a day can increase your chances of several cancers (scary but
true). It also puts you at risk for asthma and other chronic conditions.
When you last smoked makes a big difference, though, because some of
the damage reverses itself over time.

 HOW MUCH YOU DRINK: Do you really need to tell her about
that weekend cosmo habit? In a word: Yes. How much you imbibe affects
which meds your MD gives you (some cause serious side effects when
mixed with booze). It can even help her diagnose you: Drinkers bring a
different set of possibilities to the table.

YOUR OFFICE LIFE: Fact is, your job has a huge impact on your mind
and body, so it's an important clue for your doc. People who are on their
feet a lot tend to get varicose veins. Work at a computer all day? Carpal
tunnel might explain the strange loss of grip you're experiencing. Filling
your doctor in helps *her* help *you* stay well.

Q.

A few times lately, I've seen bright-red blood in the toilet. I am officially freaking out. Could I have colon cancer?

It's unlikely, but blood in your stool should always be discussed with your doctor. When you see a little bit of bright-red blood on your toilet paper or in the commode, it's usually the result of an external problem, such as an anal fissure or hemorrhoids. Anal fissures are tears in the lining of the anal canal caused by hard or large stools. More than 90 percent of these tears heal on their own within a couple of weeks, but before they heal you might see blood with a bowel movement.

The culprit could also be your diet. Everything from beets to red licorice can give your stool a crimson cast.

Straining when you're constipated can irritate an existing hemorrhoid as well, and that can cause light bleeding. Pregnant women are especially prone to hemorrhoids, and by age 50, more than half of us will have had to cope with one. Over-the-counter creams can really soothe the itching and burning, and a high-fiber diet will help prevent them from growing.

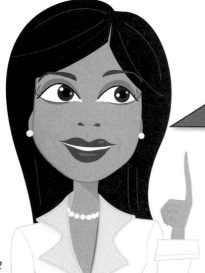

PSST, FROM DR. RAJ!
Ask for the first appointment of the day. We're fresh (as is our staff), and we haven't had time to get backed up with other patients or emergencies, so you'll get in and out quickly.

The bottom line? It's probably not cancer. But if you see blood for more than one day or notice changes in your bowel habits such as increased diarrhea or constipation, get in to see your MD. Most physicians will recommend regular colonoscopies after age 50, but if your family has a history of colon cancer or you have recurring problems, your doctor may advise you to start sooner.

• • • • • •

Q. I feel like my bladder must be shrinking. Lately I'm always looking for the nearest bathroom. What's wrong with me?

You could have a urinary tract infection. UTIs are the result of bacteria entering through the urethra and multiplying in the bladder. Women are twice as likely as men to develop at least one UTI in their lifetimes.

Blame it on our anatomy: Our urethra is shorter, so bacteria have to travel a shorter distance before they can wreak havoc, and as we age bladder tissues thin, making us more susceptible to infection. A frequent need to urinate plus pain and cloudy or bloody urine are common symptoms. Antibiotics like Levaquin or Cipro are the first line of treatment.

If a UTI isn't causing your peeing problem, it may be a side effect of a medication you're taking. If you're on an antidepressant (or diuretics for high blood pressure), or recently changed dosages, that may send you to the restroom more often, too. Your doc may change doses or prescribe a new medicine altogether to fix the problem.

Frequent urination is also an early sign of diabetes, and 25 percent of Americans who have the disease don't even know it. If your doc suspects diabetes, she'll order a series of blood tests to look at your blood sugar levels.

The Flatulent 5

Here are the most common gas-producing foods.
Don't say we didn't we warn you!

 SUGARS (real and fake). Complex sugars, found in some vegetables (such as cabbage and onions) and almost all fruits, can cause gas. But note: Artificial sweeteners, like those in fruit drinks and sodas, foods for diabetics, and gum, can also lead to excess gas.

 DAIRY. Milk contains lactose, a natural sugar that's notorious for causing tummy trouble and making us fart. If you suspect you're lactose intolerant, avoid milk products for a week or two and see if you notice relief. Over-the-counter lactase supplements, which you take before you eat, are also an option since they supply your system with the enzyme needed to digest milk.

 STARCHES. Potatoes, corn, pasta, and wheat can spell trouble. One safe starch? Rice.

 FIBER. It's good for you, but soluble fiber, found in foods like beans, peas, apples, oranges, and oat bran, can be tough to break down—and that often means gas for you.

 FIZZY drinks. Skip the sodas and other carbonated sips on important days. You can't go wrong with water.

Q. **Why does the inside of my butt suddenly feel so itchy at night?**

Since you asked: Anal itching around bedtime could mean you're infected with pinworms, a common parasite in the US that lives in the colon and creeps out at night to lay its eggs on the skin around your anus. Fortunately, it sounds much worse than it is.

12 times

That's the average number of times a person passes gas each day.

Q. **Oh Gross! How could I have caught that?**

You could have gotten them anywhere. The eggs can survive on sheets, towels, clothing, etc., and they can even fly into the air and, ugh, be swallowed! Yes, really—swallowed. It's also possible that you caught the tiny worms from eating food touched with contaminated hands. Think about that the next time you're tempted to hit the fast-food drive-through!

If you test positive for it, your doctor can give you medicine that should clear it right up.

· · · · · ·

Q. **Lately I've been incredibly gassy. Help!**

While certain foods tend to make us fart, not everyone reacts the same to "the usual suspects," which is why keeping a food diary is a great way to discover what grub troubles you. You don't have to totally eliminate these troublemakers, either. Just cut back on them, swearing them off only during those times when you would prefer to not erupt (your wedding day, for one). See The Flatulent 5 (left) for the things that bother most of us.

Q. Why do some farts smell and others don't?

Quite simply—it depends on what you ate. Not to get too technical on you, but that odor comes from small amounts of hydrogen sulfide gas released by bacteria in your intestines. These compounds contain sulfur (the same thing that gives rotten eggs their telltale stench). The more sulfur in your diet, the stinkier your gas. As you may have already figured out, the biggest offenders are meat, eggs, grains, and beer.

Decode Your Poo...

1) S-SHAPE: This is a perfectly normal shape—you're in the clear.

2) HARD, SMALL PEBBLES: You're constipated due to a lack of fiber (which adds bulk to your stool) and water (which helps move it out of your colon).

3) SUPER SKINNY: The can be from a lack of fiber or water, but it might also be from a growth (like a polyp) inside your body. See your doc if your stool doesn't return to normal in a few days.

4) LOOSE (LIKE A BOWL OF PORRIDGE): You may have an infection. If it doesn't clear up in three days, see your physician for some meds.

Beans, which are notorious for their gas-producing ability, don't usually cause smelly farts. Why's this? Well, beans contain soluble fiber (as do most fruits, bran, and peas), which doesn't break down until it reaches the large intestine. The digestion that occurs there causes the gas, but because it's past the stomach and small intestine (where all the other food you eat is broken down), there aren't any sulfur compounds for bacteria to eat. So lots of gas, but no scent.

· · · · · ·

Q. When I looked in the toilet today, my poop was tan! It's never been that color before. Should I be worried?

If your stool is tan or clay-colored for just a day or two, it's most likely related to something you ate. It will pass. If you've been taking OTC meds like Pepto-Bismol, Kaopectate, or other antidiarrheal meds, they can turn your stool this shade, too. Once these meds are all out of your system, the hue should return to normal.

But if you see beige for more than three days, there may be a lack of bile getting into your digestive tract. This could be from a blockage in your liver, pancreas, or gallbladder, so be sure to see your doctor stat.

FLOATER VS. SINKER

Poops that sink are most common, and they're totally normal. If you eat foods that produce more gas (think beans, red meat, cabbage), your stool will have more gas and will float. However, if you notice a consistent change from your normal BM to foul-smelling, greasy, floating stools, you may not be digesting fat properly. That could be a sign of celiac disease or an absorption problem. If your poop doesn't return to normal in five days, check in with your doctor.

Q. Why do my bowels go crazy after I down a big latte?

Caffeine essentially throws your bowels into hyperdrive. It's a cathartic, meaning it stimulates your colon to contract like crazy. And when your colon contracts, everything zooms through you faster. It may zip so fast that you end up with diarrhea. And if you have milk in your latte and you're one of the 60 percent of people worldwide who are lactose-intolerant, it's a double whammy. Not so pleasant for pre-10 a.m., right?

If you can't live without your latte, try switching to decaf. You'll still get your morning ritual, just without the sprint to the ladies' room.

• • • • • • •

Q. Help! Why do I feel so dry and sore when I have a bowel movement?

You're probably dehydrated. When your body doesn't have enough fluids, your poo doesn't either, making it harder to pass. And that can lead to pain and irritation.

My suggestion: Drink up! Increasing your fluids should ease the irritation. If that doesn't do the trick, try over-the-counter stool softeners, which soften the poo so it glides through your system. Also, don't be a hyper-wiper: The more you rub, the more you damage that delicate skin. Dry toilet paper can also add to the agony, so invest in higher quality (read: more expensive) paper, and moisten it with water before wiping. Better yet, use baby wipes. These strategies should bring relief and prevent future cases of itchy, irritated bum.

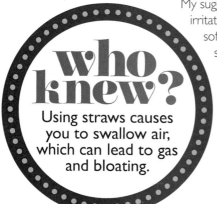

who knew?
Using straws causes you to swallow air, which can lead to gas and bloating.

4 No-Drug Ways to Stop a Stomachache

Next time you're gassy, bloated, and uncomfortable, try these natural moves.

 WALK IT OFF. Exercise might be the last thing on your mind when your stomach hurts, but a brisk 10-to-15 minute walk can do wonders. Without exercise, the intestines become sluggish, leading to cramping and constipation.

 SIP SOME TEA. Peppermint tea may help your stomach muscles relax and ease irritable bowel symptoms. But, if you have acid reflux, peppermint tea can make this worse.

PRESS HERE. Ease the stress that can trigger tummy troubles with acupressure, a proven way to release feel-good endorphins that help you relax. Try this simple trick: For 5 minutes, gently apply pressure in a circular motion with your fingers to the area that's four finger-widths above your navel.

 TAKE A BREAK. Overeating can bring on a belly-ache, so if you overdo it, just go easy the next day. Just think, if you had a muscle injury, you wouldn't push it even harder, you'd ease up. This strategy can help your digestive system bounce back. Eat smaller portions and sip lots of liquids until you feel better.

That Time of the Month

chapter

2

When you're cranky,
crampy, and craving
the whole flippin' cake

2: That Time of the Month

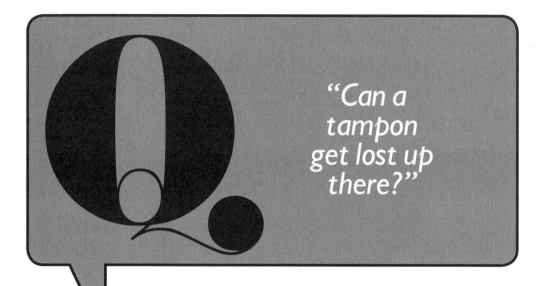

Q. "Can a tampon get lost up there?"

a Nope. A tampon can't travel beyond your vagina because your cervix blocks the way (while the cervix does have an opening, it's too small for a tampon to squeeze through). That said, that Tampax *can* move out of easy grabbing range.

So what do you do if you're searching but can't find the short string? Try this: While sitting on the toilet, bear down like you're having a bowel movement, and reach inside with your (clean) fingers. Feel around and up for the end of the tampon. If you come up empty, don't spend hours playing Where's Waldo. Instead, just call your gynecologist, and let her fish it out for you. Too embarrassed to alert your doctor? Don't be; my ob/gyn friends assure me that they take on this search mission all the time. Also, it's very easy to forget whether you have one in or not, so don't be surprised if your doc finds more than one (or none at all)!

Q. I have explosive diarrhea right around the time I get my period each month. What's wrong with me?

Absolutely nothing. It's normal to have changes in your bowel habits right around your period's arrival. Here's why: During your menstrual cycle, prostaglandins—hormone-like substances—make your uterine muscles contract, causing the cramps so many of us get "that time of the month." Sometimes these prostaglandins also trigger the smooth muscle in your intestines to contract, opening the bowel floodgates.

It helps to bulk up your stool as your period approaches: Eat more fiber-rich foods like apples, broccoli, and cauliflower. Taking ibuprofen or naproxen (with a little food) can help, but check with your doctor first because they can cause serious side effects in some people. Besides relieving other menstrual symptoms, both meds do a good job of inhibiting prostaglandin production, making you less likely to get the runs. In most cases, these moves do the trick. But if your diarrhea is very severe or prolonged, talk to your doctor about trying an antidiarrheal medication like Imodium to calm your bowels.

who knew?
The average period lasts 6 days.

• • • • • • •

Q. Why does my period smell so funky toward the end?

Benjamin Franklin famously said, "Fish and visitors smell in three days." The same goes with your monthly "visitor." At the beginning of your period, the lining of your uterus and the blood exit your body quickly (because your period is heavier), so the smell is fairly innocuous. But as the days pass, the blood and tissue in there get older; they aren't working their way out of your body as quickly. And as blood ages, it degrades—and old blood stinks. To add to the problem, the blood then sits on your pad (or if your tampon leaks, your underwear) for a few hours. Add natural sweat to the mixture, and you have a less-than-pleasant smell down there.

The simple solution: Change your pad and tampon more often (if you change it every 4 hours earlier in your cycle, aim for every 2-3 hours at the end). Showering more frequently that time of the month will also help keep the stench to a minimum. The good news is while you may notice an odor, it's doubtful anyone else will. Think about it: Have you ever noticed someone smelling of menstrual blood? I sure haven't.

• • • • • •

Q. **It seems like every time I develop a yeast infection, I have my period. Is that just a big coincidence?**

Probably not. Many women are plagued with yeast infections during their period. The culprit: a spike in the hormone progesterone—which increases during ovulation and ups the vaginal pH during your period, encouraging the growth of yeast (which is naturally present in your vagina). Some months, the yeast won't flourish beyond what the rest of your vaginal "environment" can handle. But other months, you may have one or more of those tell-tale signs of an infection—itching, burning, thick white discharge, and discomfort during sex.

Don't think you have to suffer from a yeast infection and your period at the same time, though. Treat yourself with an over-the-counter remedy (just don't use tampons); if that doesn't do the trick, see your gynecologist for a prescription for a one-day oral antifungal medication.

• • • • • •

Q. **Does an over-the-counter vaginal yeast treatment work during your period—or does the blood just dilute it?**

The treatment still works—but while you're treating your yeast problem, use pads. Tampons may absorb some of the medication, which could prevent you from getting enough to cure your problem.

Q. My flow is so heavy that even super-absorbent tampons aren't enough. Is there anything I can do?

If you need to change your tampon or pad more than every 1 to 2 hours, or if your period lasts longer than seven days, talk to your gyno about being tested for a bleeding disorder. New research shows that 25 percent of women who have a super-heavy flow may have one and not know it. Birth control pills can help regulate the bleeding by thinning out the uterine lining, and they can also help if a hormonal imbalance is the cause of the bleeding.

There is also a possibility that fibroids (which are noncancerous growths of the uterus) or polyps (growths on the inner wall of the uterus, sometimes protruding into the uterine cavity) are causing your heavy periods. If so, your gyno should be able to diagnose you.

PSST, FROM DR. RAJ!

If you have any worries at all about your PMS symptoms or period, keep a journal for a month or two of what you experience and when. Then bring it to your gyno. Your notes will help her understand exactly what's going on so she can help you find relief.

5 Foods That Fight PMS

 GREEK YOGURT: Why? It's rich in calcium, and research shows that this mineral eases PMS symptoms. Also, the probiotics can ease the tummy woes that often flare up this time of month.

 ALMONDS: Snack away! Nuts are packed with vitamin E, which helps alleviate many PMS symptoms.

 PUMPKIN SEEDS: Their secret ingredient is magnesium, a big-time bloat-buster.

 SALMON: Omega-3s are a no-drug way to ease menstrual cramps.

TURKEY: Its tryptophan can help beat irritability.

...and 3 foods that'll make you even crabbier

POTATO CHIPS: Salty snacks cause you to retain more water. Avoid 'em pre-period.

COFFEE: The caffeine can make anxiety and sleep issues worse, plus cause breasts to become tender.

CROISSANTS, SCONES, AND MUFFINS: Sugary breakfasts cause a quick release of insulin into the bloodstream that will make you feel even more down and draggy. Eat oatmeal for breakfast instead.

Q. Why am I such a lightweight right before my period? One drink, and I'm a goner!

Blame the hormone progesterone. Why? It surges during the premenstrual phase of your period, lowering your alcohol tolerance (and, incidentally, your ability to resist chocolate!).

If you are prone to PMS, it's wise to lay off the booze while you're in premenstrual mode. Not only will alcohol cause you to get drunk more quickly, but because it's a depressant, it may intensify your PMS (that means you may suffer from increased frustration, anxiety, and depression).

But even if you're not extra-moody before menstruation, consider cutting back on cocktails before your period. Why? Alcohol tends to dehydrate you, and your body needs all the fluids it can get right before your period.

· · · · · ·

Q. Everyone says women want sex most mid-cycle when they're ovulating, but I'm most turned on *during* my period. Does this mean I'm not ovulating?

Not at all. Textbooks say a woman's libido should be highest when she's ovulating. That makes sense from an evolutionary standpoint since that is when we're most likely to get pregnant, and getting pregnant ensures the survival of the species. But we all know that we are more complex than just baby-producing machines, right?

That's why many of us feel extra amorous during our periods. It could be because we're less worried about getting pregnant. Or it may be because the increase in blood flow to the pelvic region boosts sensation, making even the slightest touch feel better than pre-period. Another period perk: The blood itself is a natural lubricant.

BOTTOM LINE:
It's common to prefer period sex. And there isn't a study to suggest it means you're not ovulating regularly.

2: That Time of the Month

Q. I want to have children some day, but I have super-light periods. Does that mean I'm not ovulating?

While a light period could suggest anovulation, or lack of ovulation, it may simply mean you're blessed with a light period and have nothing to stress about (except the fact that your friends are all jealous). The only way to find out is to check for ovulation.

You can actually do this yourself with an over-the-counter ovulation kit. The test strips check your urine for a Luteinizing Hormone (LH) surge, which indicates ovulation. If you detect a spike in LH, your super-light period is just that—a super-light period. Don't see a surge or worried the test isn't working? See your gyno. She will be able to check in-office for the LH surge and, depending on what the test reveals, fill you in on your options.

• • • • • •

Q. What are the honest-to-goodness odds you'll get pregnant having unprotected sex during your period? They have to be low, right?

They are low, but not low enough to chance it. As some of us have found out, even a low chance can lead to a bouncing bundle of joy.

Every woman's cycle is different, and many of us don't have our individual schedule down to a science. Your cycle can fluctuate from month to month, making it hard to pinpoint when you're most likely to get pregnant (and not get pregnant). Another concern: Sperm can live in your body for five days, and your egg can be viable for 24 hours. If you have a short cycle, that means you definitely could get pregnant from sex during your period.

Also, some women experience spotting during the most fertile phase of their cycle and mistake it for their period. If you have unprotected sex then, your chances of getting pregnant are obviously much higher.

My advice? If you don't want to get pregnant, don't ever risk it. Instead, use protection even during your period.

NORMAL / NOT NORMAL

How can you tell normal PMS from I-need-mood-meds PMS?

 NORMAL: Feeling cranky for a day or two before your period.

 NOT NORMAL: Feeling out-of-control cranky for 10 solid days.

 NORMAL: Not being able to sleep for a night or so before your period.

NOT NORMAL: Tossing and turning every night for two weeks or longer.

 NORMAL: Feeling a little sluggish a few days before your period starts.

 NOT NORMAL: Not being able to get out of bed for a week before your period starts.

NORMAL: Being in a funk for a couple of days when you're in PMS mode.

NOT NORMAL: Suffering from feelings of total hopelessness and despair that time of the month.

NORMAL: Feeling irritated about everyday annoyances (getting cut off in traffic, your husband not taking the garbage out).

NOT NORMAL: Getting into a yelling, screaming, throwing-things rage over your husband not taking the garbage out.

NORMAL: Tearing up while watching sappy made-for-tv movies.

NOT NORMAL: Repeatedly bursting into tears and not knowing why.

2: That Time of the Month

Q. Is it normal for my boobs to get a whole cup-size bigger during PMS? It's such a dramatic change that I need two different sets of bras!

Yep, breast inflation is completely normal. During the premenstrual phase, we have higher levels of the hormones progesterone and prolactin, both of which can cause breast tissue to swell and milk glands to increase in size. Plus, our bodies retain water during that premenstrual period. The change in boob size varies from woman to woman and sometimes from month to month. Some women won't notice much difference in their ta-tas, while others get a monthly (temporary) boob job.

Though you can't stop this hormonal process, there are things you can do to make your PMS breast makeover less pronounced. To keep water retention in check, cut back on your salt intake. Keep an eye out for hidden sodium in soup, vegetable juice, and fast food. If that doesn't help, water pills can help with the water retention. If the change is dramatic and it really stresses you out, talk to your doctor about going on oral contraceptives. By regulating the hormonal fluctuation, the Pill can help keep you in one cup-size all month long.

· · · · · ·

who knew?

The Japanese term for that time of the month is **"Ichigo-chan."** Translation? Little Miss Strawberry!

Q. Sometimes when I take over-the-counter period medicine, I feel like my heart's beating out of my chest. Why does it affect me like that?

Some PMS or menstrual meds contain caffeine to help the symptoms of fatigue and bloating (caffeine is a diuretic, meaning it flushes out extra fluids). A two-caplet dose of some of these products gives you the same caffeine jolt as a cup of coffee! If you're not a caffeine drinker or you know you're sensitive to this stimulant, check the label of any PMS meds before using them. Better yet, if you need the pain relief but don't want the caffeine, try a nonsteroidal anti-inflammatory drug (NSAID) like ibuprofen or naproxen.

If you do decide to take the PMS meds, just limit your caffeine intake from other sources (coffee, tea, chocolate) while you're on it so you don't turn into a ball of jitters.

● ● ● ● ● ●

Q. How long can you leave a tampon in without catching something nasty? Sometimes I forget and leave it in all day long!

I wouldn't go pushing my luck on this one. You should really change your tampon every 4 to 6 hours. Leaving one in longer can cause vaginal irritation with the possibility of infection. The most serious one you can develop is toxic shock syndrome (TSS), a potentially life-threatening bacterial infection usually caused by *Staphylococcus aureus* (Staph). TSS can develop suddenly, and its symptoms include a high fever, vomiting or diarrhea, low blood pressure, and seizures. If you have these symptoms, go straight to the emergency room. If you delay, the infection and accompanying low blood pressure can lead to kidney failure.

Now does that mean it's a huge problem if you stretch that time frame? Not always. In fact, we probably all know women who have forgotten tampons for several days and lived to tell about it. But there is the potential for a very serious infection, so get in the habit of swapping out tampons on a regular basis and sleeping in pads rather than tampons.

HOW **BAD** IS IT REALLY?

To pop three Advil for super bad cramps

If you don't have a previous history of stomach ulcers, it's okay to take three ibuprofen, such as Advil, once in a while. Three Advil (600 milligrams of ibuprofen) is actually a prescription-strength dosage, so it won't hurt you in the short term. But if you're taking Advil or one of its sister meds like Motrin daily for more than three or four days, even two at a time, can cause stomach inflammation or ulcers. To help prevent stomach damage, always take these pills with food. And if you find yourself regularly reaching for three ibuprofen pills to ease your cramps, talk to your gynecologist about whether you should be on a prescription-strength medication.

BY THE NUMBERS

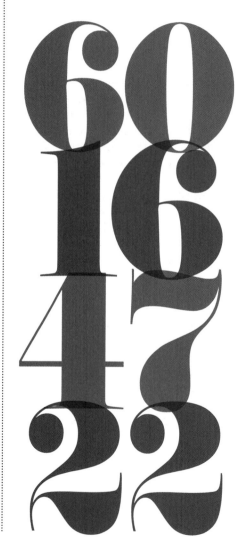

60% of women have had unprotected sex during their period.

. . . .

16% of women have left a tampon in for 24 hours or longer.

. . . .

47% of women have had cramps so bad they called in sick to work.

. . . .

22% of women say that their most embarrassing moment was forgetting to put in a tampon.

. . . .

Source: Health.com poll

Q. I can't stop yawning before I get my period. Why?

You're not alone on this. Seventy-five percent of women report symptoms of PMS, with fatigue being one of the most common complaints they have. It's probably due to the fluctuation of hormone/chemical levels—particularly progesterone, estrogen, and serotonin. There are a few things you can do that'll help you feel more alert.

First, keep up your exercise routine. I know, I know—it's tempting to slack off when you're feeling pooped. But exercise boosts your natural endorphins and helps reduce premenstrual symptoms. It's also a good idea to eat whole grains like oatmeal, brown rice, and popcorn (minus the butter and salt) to keep your blood sugar steady throughout the whole day. When your blood sugar is on an even keel, you'll feel less sluggish. Skip the sugary snacks; they cause an almost-instant blood sugar surge and then an even more sudden crash.

So exhausted you can't even get out of bed? You may have the more severe, sometimes-debilitating premenstrual dysphoric disorder (PMDD): About 10 percent of menstruating women are thought to have it. If you suspect you have it (find out more on page 39, other symptoms include persistent anger or irritability; feeling completely overwhelmed; flu-like symptoms like achy muscles, headaches, and joint pain; and drastic changes in appetite—like overeating or lack of appetite), see your doctor. She can diagnose you and help you find the best treatment, be it antidepressants to control serotonin levels or an oral contraceptive to stabilize the hormone fluctuations.

GOT BAD CRAMPS?

Pinch either side of your foot in the groove under and slightly behind the anklebone.

Then take your other hand and firmly press the center of the big toe on the same foot. This reflexology move is believed to relax the ovaries and uterus, as well as the hypothalamus gland, which helps regulate hormones.

2: That Time of the Month

Q. Why do I crave chocolate like crazy right before getting my period?

Honestly? We have no clue. (We don't know why many PMS symptoms happen!) Lots of theories exist, and the best ones seem to point to—you guessed it—hormones.

The good news is we do know how to keep these cravings from ruling your life. Though your body may be crying out for a box of Mallomars, you're better off resisting the sweet stuff.

Too many sugary treats cause your blood sugar to spike and then plummet. As soon as it crashes, you'll be reaching for more cookies. This cycle can lead to low energy and weight gain. Instead, choose complex carbs like fruits, vegetables, nuts, and grains (whole grains preferably). These treats keep your blood sugar at a somewhat-even level all day long, preventing you from feeling cranky and craving more candy.

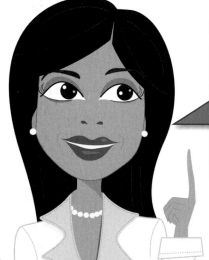

PSST, FROM DR. RAJ!
I've found that exercise really helps ease the physical and emotional symptoms of PMS, including irritability, low energy, and bloating. The key is to work out at least 30 minutes, three times a week.

Can't wish away that sweet craving? Grab a square or two of dark chocolate instead of the giant bag of M&Ms. Keep a bar in the freezer so you have it when you're in PMS mode. Not only will you satisfy your sweet tooth, but you'll also help your health: Dark chocolate is heart-healthy, thanks to its protective antioxidants. Now that's killing two birds with one stone!

· · · · · ·

Q. Why does my sweat smell worse before I get my period?

Fluctuations in progesterone make you sweat more from the apocrine glands—those in your armpits, scalp, and genitals. Sweat itself doesn't actually smell. But bacteria on the surface of the skin love to feed on sweat (what we identify as the smell of sweat is really the smell of bacterial breakdown). So the more you perspire, the more there is for bacteria to feast on, making your sweat stinkier.

Q. Anything I can do about it?

Keep the growth of bacteria at a minimum by taking daily showers. And be sure to hit the shower immediately after a workout to get rid of the sweat. As soon as you get out of the shower, apply an antiperspirant-deodorant, and do it again right before bedtime. These moves will help stop the odor before it starts. If the smell continues to bug you, see your doctor for a prescription-strength antiperspirant.

HOW **BAD** IS IT *REALLY?*

To have only four periods a year

With new birth control options, we don't have to have monthly periods. We can even have as few as four safely because when you're on birth control, you're not ovulating. So the fact that you're not having monthly periods isn't meaningful in any way. No ovulation, no need to have a period.

NOT TO WORRY!

Many women have irregular periods

Stress, illness, and changes in medication can make your period come early, late, or not at all. If you're late by more than a week or if you have consistently random periods though, see your gyno.

Q. Sometimes my period looks extra clotty and like there's tissue attached to it (gross, right?). What could that be?

That stuff that looks like tissue? It is tissue. But don't worry—it's not a bad sign.

Each month, when your cycle starts, your uterus prepares for a possible pregnancy by thickening its lining, also known as the endometrium. Mid-cycle, you ovulate—your ovaries produce an egg, and this egg travels down the fallopian tube. If that egg runs into sperm, it becomes fertilized, and you get pregnant! If not, your body realizes you're not pregnant and sloughs off (or sheds) the lining of the uterus—the endometrium. This is what you're seeing in your menstrual blood.

So it's totally normal to see clumps of tissue. The amount of tissue will vary from woman to woman and sometimes month to month. That means you may notice a bunch one month and almost nothing the next.

• • • • • •

Q. Is it true you should avoid yoga during your period?

For years, some yogis have said that inverted poses like shoulder stands create an obstruction to the natural energy of the menstrual flow, which is, of course, downward—and their students have dutifully passed this info along. But there are no medical studies or research supporting the advice to avoid inversions—or any other yoga pose—while you have your period.

The best rule of thumb is to do what feels comfortable to you. If an inversion doesn't sound appealing, by all means skip it. But if it does, then go for it. You may find that some common poses like cat and cobra actually alleviate PMS-induced cramps and moodiness. Ask your yoga instructor for pointers on how to do these moves and others that relieve period-related symptoms like low energy, lower back pain, and more.

4 Things Mom Was Right About

 CHICKEN SOUP EASES A COLD. Yep—it has anti-inflammatory properties that relieve sore throats and stuffy noses.

 A LITTLE SUN IS HEALTHY. It helps your body make vitamin D, a bone-booster that may cut your risk of some cancers.

 CARROTS ARE GREAT FOR YOUR EYES. They contain beta-carotene, which gets converted to vitamin A, which is essential for eye health.

 SODA WILL ROT YOUR TEETH. The acids, not the sugar, eat away at tooth enamel.

And 2 Things She Got Wrong

Though we know she meant well...

 READING IN DIM LIGHT WILL MAKE YOU GO BLIND.

 IF YOU GO OUTSIDE WITH WET HAIR, YOU'LL CATCH A COLD.

The Girls

chapter 3

Yes, we all obsess about our breasts!

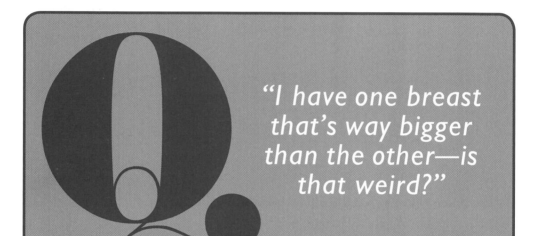

"I have one breast that's way bigger than the other—is that weird?"

Nope. Most women have slight differences in the shape and size of their breasts (one nipple points north, while the other points south, for example). It's normal to have one breast larger than the other—sometimes even by a cup size or two. I know women who affectionately refer to one breast as "the big sister" and the other as "the scrawny one." If you really look at people closely, you'll notice that most of us have minor asymmetry in our bodies—our two eyes or ears aren't exactly the same, for example. So it makes sense that we'd also have some asymmetry in our boobs.

As long as this size difference isn't new, you're okay. But if one breast has suddenly gotten bigger or feels different (thicker, fuller, or lumpy), you need to be checked out by your doc. A unilateral (one-sided) change could be a sign of a cyst or even a tumor.

Q. Why are my nipples pink but my best friend's are brown?

The hue of your nipples—just like your hair and eye color—is determined by genetics. Most darker-skinned ethnicities have darker nipples, but many Caucasian women also have brown nipples.

Nipples and areola (the skin around the nipple) also darken as we age and while we are pregnant or breastfeeding. If it's a pregnancy-induced color change, your nipples should return to their original shade after you've finished breastfeeding.

• • • • • •

Q. My boobs are naturally lumpy—how will I know when I have a bad one?

That's a good question. Lumpy breasts, or fibrocystic breasts, is a very common benign (noncancerous) condition, but it does present a challenge. Women like you have more dense areas of tissue in their breasts than other women, so mammograms aren't as effective a screen for breast cancer. Your doctor may recommend an ultrasound test in addition or instead.

Our breasts tend to get lumpier right before our period, so when you do your self-exams (or when you're scheduling a mammo or an ob/gyn appointment), it's best to do it right after your period. If you notice a new lump that lasts one menstrual cycle, or if it feels different than others (hard or closer to the surface of your skin), be sure to get it checked out. But don't panic: 80 percent of breasts lumps are benign. This question reminds me to remind you: Get to know your breasts. Make sure to schedule yearly checkups and annual screenings after age 40…or earlier if you have a family history of breast cancer. (Yep, despite the fact that the guidelines have recently changed, I still urge women to get annual mammograms after 40.) And feel yourself up regularly: Do informal self-exams once a month so that if something new pops up, you'll know.

Q. My mom and sister are a cup-size E and D; both of my grandmothers had very large breasts, too. Yet I'm only an A cup. Did I miss out on the boob gene?

Yep, you may have. Breast size is mostly determined by genetics, so you're right to wonder about this. But strange as it seems, you can actually inherit your chest size from your dad. Is he from A-cup stock? If so, that's your answer.

Another theory: If you're thin but your mom, sis, and grandmas are all overweight, their triple-Ds may be due to excess pounds, not genetics. In any case, don't sweat your size. There are many women who'd kill to be able to rock a cute tank top (sans bra to boot!).

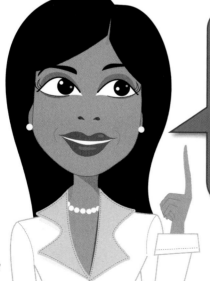

PSST, FROM DR. RAJ!
Sleeping on your chest can actually change the shape of your breasts over time, stretching the skin and leading to sagging. So to preserve what you've got, sleep on your side with breasts supported by a pillow.

Q. Is it true that my underwire bra will give me breast cancer?

Not true! There was once a theory that underwire bras blocked the lymphatic drainage of the breast, causing an accumulation of toxins that could then lead to cancer. But lots of studies have looked for a link between underwire bras and cancer and haven't found a problem. Plus, we now know that blocked lymphatic drainage *doesn't* lead to breast cancer. So keep on wearing your favorite underwire bra; it's completely safe.

• • • • • •

Q. I just noticed a tiny growth of what looks like extra skin under my left breast. Could it be cancer?

It's more likely a skin tag, a common and harmless type of growth that tends to first pop up in your 30s, often on the neck, underarms, groin, eyelids, or yes, beneath the breasts. Skin tags are caused by chafing and irritation from skin rubbing together. They may also be caused by hormones since many women notice they have more skin tags during and after pregnancy. A dermatologist or primary care doc can easily remove an annoying skin tag either by snipping it off with scissors (don't try this at home!) or with liquid nitrogen or medical cauterization. Your insurance may even cover it, but check first.

Skin tags shouldn't cause pain (unless they're in an area where they can get caught in a zipper—yeow).

If you want a reassuring second opinion, have it checked out by your doctor or dermatologist. Final note: If the spot in question oozes or bleeds, it probably isn't a skin tag, so see your doc ASAP to rule out skin cancer.

NORMAL OR NOT:
Stretch marks on your boobs
Normal
You can develop stretch marks anywhere you gain and lose weight—breasts included. It's common for these to pop up post-pregnancy. Your breasts grow dramatically during those months, and once that weight is gone you can be left with an unwanted souvenir. Whether you get them is mostly due to your genes, alas, so don't waste a drop of cash on expensive creams that claim to prevent them.

HOW **BAD** IS IT REALLY?

To go braless

It's not so bad. There's no research showing that bra-skipping leads to faster sagging (we're all headed south at one speed or another). However, when your breasts are very full (like when you're lactating) or large, letting your girls hang out increases your risk of neck or back pain. So in these cases, you should always wear a supportive bra. Also, it's absolutely crucial to wear a good sports bra when you're exercising, especially if you have larger breasts. All that bouncing up and down can stretch your breast ligaments, and stretched ligaments *do* make you sag. A supportive bra keeps you perky by holding ligaments in place while you work out.

Q. I noticed a few hairs on my chest. Help!

Don't worry, you're not alone. Many women have hirsutism—a condition where hair appears in typically male hair-growth areas: the face (beard or mustache), chest, or back.

If you have a lot of unwanted hair (or it seems to crop up in lots of places), pay a visit to your doctor. She may want to test you for a hormonal imbalance (like polycystic ovary syndrome), which can cause unusual hair growth. If you test positive, your doc will prescribe medication to treat it (bye-bye, breast hair). Some medicines, such as steroids and certain drugs used to treat endometriosis, can also cause hair growth. If an Rx is the culprit, switching meds or changing dosages should solve the problem. Of course, some women are just genetically predisposed to sprouting extra hair. Fortunately, there are now great removal options. What's best? Depends on how much money, time, and pain you're willing to put in:

- **Shaving** is easy and super-cheap (just the cost of shaving cream and razors). However, you'll have to continue shaving as the hair grows back.
- **Plucking** is free (minus the cost of the tweezers), but a lot of women say it takes too much time and they can't stand the torture of pulling each hair one by one. Results last two to three weeks.
- **Waxing** is fairly inexpensive, depending on the surface area you're waxing. But if you can't stomach the idea of having a stranger rip out your hair (or torturing yourself in this manner), move on. Results usually last three to four weeks.
- **Depilatories** (aka hair-removal creams) get the job done, and they're cheap (about $5 in drugstores). They

work by breaking down the hair's proteins, disintegrating the hair. You spread a thick layer of the cream over the area, let it sit for a few minutes, and then wipe away. Downside: Some women find the smell repulsive. Results typically last two weeks.

- **Bleaching** the hairs so they're less noticeable is also an option. But before bleaching the whole area, do a test patch to make sure you don't react. Be sure to use bleach products that are designed for the face and body, not your head, because they're less likely to irritate your skin. Mix according to the directions, and apply it to a small area, wiping it off after the designated time. If in 24 hours you don't notice any redness or burning, go for it. However, if you feel burning or itching while the product is on your skin, take it right off and move on to another hair-zapping method. Results will last about two weeks, depending on how fast your hair grows.

- **Electrolysis,** which uses heat energy to destroy the growth center of hair follicles, may be your best bet for permanent hair removal. It can be expensive (around $100 per hour), and the larger the surface, the more time it takes. An upper lip, say, may take an hour.

- **Laser hair removal** is also worth considering, especially if you're looking for a somewhat-permanent option. It requires multiple trips to your derm (don't trust a medi spa; see a board-certified dermatologist), as well as a good amount of cash (a single laser treatment can run as much as $350 and rarely, if ever, will insurance cover it). Laser heat is used to inflame the hair follicle, leaving it dormant and unable to produce hair. You'll feel warmth on your skin during the treatment, and since hair follicles are surrounded by nerve endings, you might feel some pain when they get inflamed from the laser. Most people require three to seven treatments, spaced a month or two apart. To keep an area completely smooth, you may need maintenance sessions about once a year (more or less often depending on your hair—everyone is different).

NOT TO WORRY:
Nipple hair is the norm

Every woman has between 2 and 15 dark, straight strands growing. You can wax or tweeze 'em if they bug you.

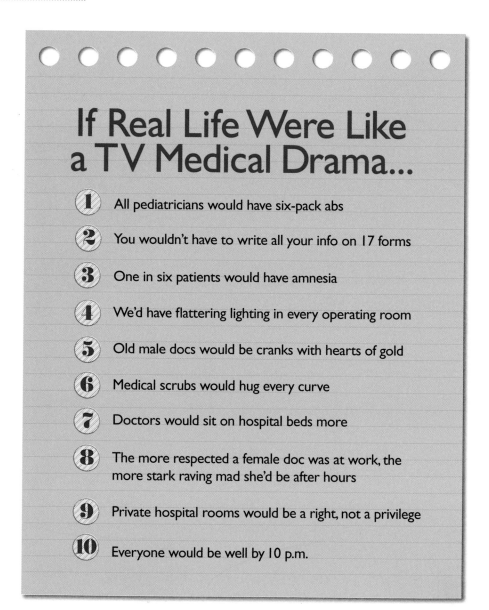

If Real Life Were Like a TV Medical Drama...

1. All pediatricians would have six-pack abs

2. You wouldn't have to write all your info on 17 forms

3. One in six patients would have amnesia

4. We'd have flattering lighting in every operating room

5. Old male docs would be cranks with hearts of gold

6. Medical scrubs would hug every curve

7. Doctors would sit on hospital beds more

8. The more respected a female doc was at work, the more stark raving mad she'd be after hours

9. Private hospital rooms would be a right, not a privilege

10. Everyone would be well by 10 p.m.

Q. No matter how much I bathe, the area under my breasts is red and smelly. What is going on?

This sounds like intertrigo, or inflammation in the body's folds. Trapped moisture or chafing from skin rubbing together—armpits, between legs, under the belly, and beneath the breasts—can lead to a bacterial or fungal infection. Heavy people are most at risk, but women with large breasts can also develop this pesky problem.

You can't scrub it away—and you may irritate the already-sensitive skin. Instead, talk to your doctor about an antibacterial or antifungal cream. You can speed up healing and prevent another outbreak. First, if you're overweight, drop some pounds. Wear cotton and breathable fabrics to wick away moisture. A supportive bra (with wide straps and three hooks across in back) helps keep your breasts from dragging against your skin. Dry the area under your chest well after your bath or shower. Tip: Use a blow dryer (on cool, of course) to gently dry off problem zones.

60% of women have worried because one breast looks different than the other.

Source: Health.com poll

● ● ● ● ● ● ●

Q. It looks like I have a second nipple on one boob—is that possible?

Actually, yes. This is called a supernumerary nipple—a third nipple. Between 1 and 5 percent of people (women and men) are born with them. They can be tiny (like a mole) or large and function like a regular nipple. They can have breast tissue around them and resemble a mini breast. These third nipples grow along the "milk lines" in your body (imagine a straight line from your armpit to your groin, passing through your nipples) and are typically directly beneath one of the nipples on your breasts. If you're lactating, they can (in rare cases) produce milk.

A third nipple is 100 percent harmless. But if, for cosmetic reasons, you'd like to have it removed, you can see a plastic surgeon.

Q. I'm thinking about getting fake boobs. Any risks I should know about?

As with any surgery, there's a possibility of infection, bleeding, and reactions to anesthesia or pain medicines. But with breast augmentation, there's also a risk you'll develop scar tissue that can distort the shape of your breast and have an implant leak or rupture, which requires additional surgery to fix. And here's a little secret you don't often hear: You're committing to a lifetime of surgery—you have to have implants redone about every 10 years or so. Also consider whether you hope to breastfeed. Breast augmentation surgery can damage nerves, milk ducts, and glands, making it impossible to breastfeed. Also know that if you ever opt to have your implants removed, your breasts won't return to their original form: The surgery permanently changes the look of your natural breasts. So be sure to ask your doctor lots of questions, and carefully weigh all the pros and cons before you make the final call.

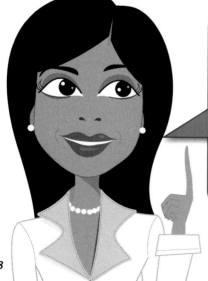

PSST, FROM DR. RAJ!
Make your next appointment with your doctor before you walk out the door. It's easy to say you'll call and then forget. Studies show you're more likely to actually have that follow-up if you schedule it before you leave your doc's office.

Q. I have huge nipples! It's so embarrassing because I always have the dreaded "headlights" look.

Poor thing. Even those of us with smaller nips know how you feel—there's nothing more maddening than seeming like you're flaunting your body when you'd actually give anything to have your body stand out less. This may make you feel better: Nipples come in all sizes, and they're all normal. As you probably know, all nipples swell and become erect when we're sexually aroused. This natural process also happens when the tiny muscles around the nipples are stimulated—by cold or from something rubbing them (like a shirt or bra). In addition to having more prominent nipples, you may be more sensitive than other women to these stimuli.

The best solution: new padded bras. They work wonders, preventing unwanted stimulation from your bra or shirt and helping conceal your bumps. Also, wearing thicker fabrics like cotton makes it harder for the headlights to shine through.

• • • • • •

Q. How much sagging is normal? I feel like my breasts are heading south faster than my friends'!

As we get older the ligaments that hold up our breasts lose their elasticity—the ability to bounce back to their original shape or size after being stretched. Plus, breast tissue becomes more fatty and tends to have less shape and perkiness, which leads to more sag. Weight gain or loss, pregnancy, and breastfeeding all contribute, too, because when the breasts enlarge and then shrink, the skin doesn't snap back. Things to do that help: Wear a super-supportive bra, especially when exercising. Look for one that has a thick back with at least three hooks. Regular exercise is important, because it improves skin and ligament elasticity. Also, avoid yo-yo dieting because that leads to stretched skin and the inevitable sag. And hey, if you *really* hate the way yours look, plastic surgery is always an option.

Q. I have deep stabbing pain in my breasts. Could it be cancer?

You can rest easy: Breast pain is not a common symptom of cancer. Instead, I can think of a couple of more likely causes of your pain.

Are you breastfeeding? You may have a bacterial infection of the breast called mastitis, which sometimes causes fever and always needs to be treated urgently with antibiotics. (It's possible but rare to have it when you're not breastfeeding.) And, it's also possible your baby has *Oropharyngeal candidiasis*, or more simply, thrush. Thrush is a yeast infection in your baby's mouth that leaves white patches on her mouth and tongue. You can tell these white patches from traces of breast milk or formula because they can't be wiped away. While nursing, your little one can pass this infection

Decode Your Nipple Discharge

Leaking? Here's a guide to what might be up. Call your gyno about any discharge that lasts longer than a day or two.

YELLOW: This can be normal. Or it might be a sign of fibrocystic breast disease or infection.

MILKY: If you're lactating, it's normal. Milky discharge can also signal stimulation of milk ducts, increased prolactin levels, or pregnancy.

GREEN: This too can be normal, or it might suggest fibrocystic breast disease or infection.

BLOODY: This is rarely okay. It could be due to a benign growth, called a papilloma, or a breast injury. If you have bloody discharge, see your doctor as soon as possible.

to you, giving you a yeast infection in—of all places—your breasts and/or nipples. You'll likely feel stabbing pain in your breasts, especially while breastfeeding.

It's not serious, but you need to see your ob/gyn. Both you and baby need to be treated with an antifungal cream such as nystatin (applied to your infant's mouth and your breasts and nipples). It's crucial that you clean your nipples thoroughly after every feeding to prevent passing the yeast back and forth.

Not breastfeeding? Another possibility is mastalgia, a very common condition that may be related to your cycle (cyclical pain) or not (noncyclical). If your discomfort isn't tied to your cycle, the problem may be a nearby muscle or a cyst. If you have cyclical mastalgia, though, the pain is linked to hormonal fluctuation and will likely begin or worsen around the time of ovulation and continue until the start of your period. It might be more severe in one breast and vary from month to month.

Try wearing looser-fitting clothing around the time of the month when you feel the pain. If the pain is unbearable or gets worse over time, see your doctor—she'll want to rule out blocked glands or a tumor.

• • • • • •

Q. Who is more likely to get breast cancer: someone who is flat-chested or really curvy?

Being well-endowed doesn't up your chances of developing cancer. That said, being overweight *does* increase your risk of breast cancer (and other health problems). So if your curves are from added weight, you're at a higher risk than a woman who is slim. (Obesity raises your risk of many cancers, so it's important to try to reach and maintain a healthy weight.)

Big boobs can make feeling lumps or detecting tumors more difficult, for sure. Larger breasts have more tissue, and the more tissue there is, the more you have to feel and inspect. That's why it's important for women with larger breasts to visit their doctor annually (if not more often) for a clinical breast exam and get yearly mammograms if over 40.

Between the Sheets

chapter

4

Warning: This chapter goes there!

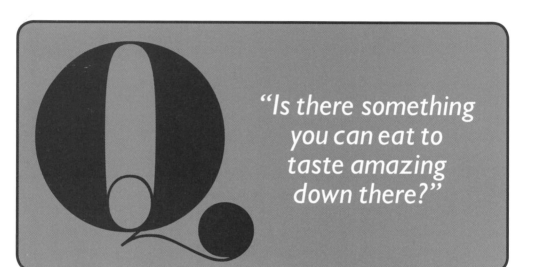

"Is there something you can eat to taste amazing down there?"

Well, I don't know about amazing, but there are some things that will make you taste lighter—or better, if you will. Take a cue from your vegetarian friends: Fruits and vegetables like pineapple and celery give your vaginal fluids a milder taste. Meat, fish, and dairy products, on the other hand, make them taste stronger. So do garlic, spices, and caffeine. Drinking a lot of water actually helps flush out any possible offenders. Using flavored lubricants is another way to lighten the taste. Just make sure they don't stray too far into the vagina, where they can irritate you.

Q. Is it true that some women just smell fishier? How do I know if I do?

A word about vaginal odor: All women have it. It's completely natural and not something to stress about. In fact, most men consider that scent arousing.

That said, if you notice that you smell unusually fishy or your odor is particularly strong post-sex or after washing your vagina with soap, you might have bacterial vaginosis or BV—an easily treatable infection caused by an imbalance of the normal vaginal bacteria. You should see your gynecologist, who can test for it and, if you come up positive, prescribe an antibiotic that should clear it up. One final note: While BV isn't a sexually transmitted disease (STD), vaginal odor can sometimes be a sign of one, so your gynecologist may want to rule out that, too.

17% of women have eaten something special to smell better down there.
Source: Health.com poll

• • • • • • •

Q. Anything I can do to prevent getting a vaginal infection like BV?

Some habits definitely up your odds. Here are three healthy moves to help you steer clear:

Don't douche. You may have heard this before, but your vagina is self-cleaning, so there's no need to ever douche. Doing so can actually disrupt the natural harmony of your vaginal flora and put you at risk for another unpleasant infection.

Wear all-cotton undies. The all-cotton kind let the air flow better than synthetics and keep moisture (which breeds bacteria) to a minimum. If you're prone to BV or yeast infections, it's also wise to swear off thongs.

Sleep commando. Forgoing panties at night helps air out your vagina, making it harder for bacteria to multiply and set up shop.

Q. Can I catch his cold from going down on him?

We catch the viruses that cause the common cold by breathing in airborne droplets or touching our noses or mouths with contaminated fingers (think shared door handles). So technically, just performing oral sex on him shouldn't get you sick. But if he touched his penis with germy hands, and then you put your mouth there, you could definitely come down with the sniffles.

In general, being in close contact with someone who has a cold ups your chances of inhaling some of their virus, so if you can't afford to get sick at the moment, keep things strictly platonic until your guy is feeling better.

· · · · · ·

Q. Can he catch my cold from going down on me?

Same story here: He won't get it from being down there, but if you've touched your vagina with contaminated hands, he could very well pick up your virus from oral sex. My advice? No getting hot and heavy while one of you is hot and sneezy.

PSST, FROM DR. RAJ!
Before you leave your doc's office, find out when and how you'll get test results. Each doctor's office has a different policy, so don't assume that no news is good news.

Q. I had sex while I had a yeast infection. Could I have passed it on to my man?

It's possible, but not likely. Yeast infections don't generally spread from person to person. We get one when there's an overgrowth of the yeast that's normally present in our own genital area. What causes yeast to multiply? Antibiotics (because they kill the good down-there bacteria that keep this fungus in check), a depressed immune system, and a warm, damp groin (from too-tight clothes, say, or synthetic fabrics).

But let's say you have loads of yeast and then have sex. You could spread the yeast to his penis. If he notices itching and redness, he should see his doctor and get a prescription antifungal treatment. While yeast infections are generally mild in men, he needs to zap it because if he doesn't, he'll just ping-pong it back to you.

HERE'S MY TIP:

Next time you have a yeast infection, skip intercourse, which can irritate you even more, cause you to pass the infection to your man (prolonging the agony for both of you), and push most of the yeast-treatment cream out, rendering it useless.

TRUE OR FALSE?
Women get blue balls, too

Half truth. For both men and women, blood flow to the genital area increases during sexual arousal. This can cause a feeling of heaviness or pressure, which goes by the unsexy term pelvic vasocongestion. It's usually relieved by orgasm, but if a woman doesn't climax, she might feel mild discomfort. It is usually short-lived and not a big deal…or at least not as big of a deal as some guys make it out to be!

· · · · · · ·

Q. Can he thrust so hard he does damage in there?

Even if the sex gets a little rough, he probably won't do any serious damage. But the friction from his penis rubbing against your vagina could cause abrasions or tears in the delicate vaginal tissue, which is no fun.

You're more likely to suffer from this unpleasant side effect if you're dry, so

HOW **BAD** IS IT *REALLY?*

To need a glass of wine to have sex

It's not the worst thing in the world. Alcohol takes away many of the inhibitions we feel when sober (you may have noticed). This is especially true when we're out of our element and not completely comfortable (the way we feel with a new partner, say). So if a glass of Pinot is what it takes to get past some normal jitters or to relax and reconnect with your man at the end of a crazy-busy day, that's totally fine. But it's a red flag if you need to knock back several drinks to ever feel up for sex. Also problematic: using booze to numb feelings of insecurity about your body or performance. Just keep in mind that alcohol decreases your sensations during sex, making it harder to reach the big O.

make sure you're fully aroused before moving on to the main event. Add lube as an extra precaution. If you feel any pain or discomfort while he's thrusting, slow him down to prevent more damage. Naturally, if it hurts a lot, stop the action completely. And if you experience pain or bleeding post-romp, take a sex sabbatical until everything has healed. Otherwise, you risk more pain and permanent scarring.

· · · · · ·

Q. Is semen fattening?

Not at all. The average ejaculate is about the size of a teaspoon. It contains sperm, sugars, and proteins—and only about 7 calories. You'll burn all those calories (and more) just rolling in the hay.

· · · · · ·

Q. If I have a cold sore and go down on him, can I give him herpes?

Okay, let's break this down because it can be confusing. There are two types of herpes. Cold sores (or oral herpes) are very common and are usually caused by Herpes Simplex 1 (HSV-1), while genital herpes are somewhat rarer and usually caused by Herpes Simplex 2 (HSV-2).

But you can get HSV-1 (aka cold sores) on your genitals and HSV-2 ("genital" herpes) in the mouth. So yes, you could spread herpes to your partner during oral sex. Your best bet: Hold off on the oral action at least until the sore has disappeared. Technically you can still transfer the herpes anytime, even when there isn't an outbreak, so the only really safe move is to have oral sex with a condom or dental dam.

Q. The condom slipped off him during sex. He fished it out, but do I have to worry about pregnancy?

You sure do. If the condom breaks or slips off, the sperm are free to go looking for an egg to fertilize.

So if you don't want to get pregnant, talk to your doctor ASAP about the morning-after pill. This treatment is available over the counter, but there are a few different types, so ask your doc which one is best for you.

Also, since condoms are not foolproof (as you now know), you may want to also ask your doctor about backup birth control. It sounds like a hassle, but if you really want to avoid pregnancy, it's smart to use two forms of protection.

43% of women have had a condom come off during sex.

Source: Health.com poll

• • • • • • •

Q. This is embarrassing, but he wants to use the back door—can that cause GI problems?

Whenever a patient asks me this question (and yep, I've heard even this one before), I say this: Anal sex usually isn't a problem. But there are some potential concerns you need to be aware of before green-lighting this request.

Because the anal sphincter is tight and there is less lubrication in the anus (it doesn't produce the natural lubrication your vagina does), anal intercourse could cause tiny abrasions, or tears, in the anus. Also, stool bacteria are present so there's a chance those abrasions and tears may become infected.

MY ADVICE:

Use lots and lots of lube. Plus, if this is a newer partner, don't forget the condom. Though you won't get pregnant this way, STDs can be transmitted through anal sex. Also, empty your bowels beforehand. And have your partner wash his penis before going from anal to vaginal sex and vice versa.

Q. I have orgasms all the time—when I'm at the gym working out or just sitting at my desk. Am I a freak?

Lucky girl! Many women have trouble having orgasms at all, and here you are having them all the time—life isn't fair!

But seriously, spontaneous orgasms (those without direct genital stimulation) are not uncommon. Some women get them by thinking erotic thoughts. Others have them while doing things that indirectly stimulate the genital area, like riding a bike, tightening pelvic muscles (like when holding in pee), sneezing, etc. Some antidepressants can cause this happy side effect, though the effect usually wears off a few weeks after starting the meds.

Don't want to peak in public? If your climaxes are a result of friction (like during a workout), double up on your underwear or wear a pad to desensitize the area.

• • • • • • •

Q. Sometimes when I'm getting hot and heavy, I'll suddenly let out a vaginal fart. How mortifying!

I guarantee this has happened to almost every woman at some point in her life, and it's mortifying. But it has nothing to do with you or your vagina; it's just a natural by-product of intercourse. During sex, air flows into the spaces around your genitals, especially any new spaces that are created from your vaginal tissues moving around as you get aroused. Sometimes, when these pockets of air escape, it makes what sounds like a fart. This air has had no contact with your colon, so there's no odor.

What can you do to avoid having a flatulent you-know-what? Use plenty of lube. Also, avoid doggie style: It causes a lot of air to flow in, upping your odds of letting loose with an embarrassing noise.

who knew?

The clitoris has **8,000** nerve endings, which is twice as many as the penis.

7 Reasons to Have Sex (and Lots of It)

 1 IT KEEPS COLDS AWAY. Having sex once or twice a week has been linked with higher levels of an antibody called immunoglobulin A or IgA, which can protect you from getting colds and other infections.

 2 IT EASES STRESS. Sex lowers blood pressure and reduces overall stress, according to Scottish research.

 3 IT KEEPS YOU SLIM. Depending on how acrobatic you are, 30 minutes of sex burns 55 calories or more. It may not sound like much, but it adds up.

4 IT HELPS YOUR HEART. While we've all seen movies where an old man has a heart attack while getting his groove on in bed, the truth is having sex twice or more a week can actually reduce the risk of a fatal heart attack.

 5 IT HELPS YOU SLEEP. The oxytocin released during orgasm also promotes sleep, according to research.

 6 IT KEEPS YOU FIT BELOW THE BELT. Doing a few pelvic-floor muscle exercises known as Kegels during sex offers a couple of benefits: You will enjoy more pleasure, and you'll also strengthen the muscles and minimize the risk of incontinence later in life.

7 IT HELPS YOU LIVE LONGER. Many experts, such as Dr. Oz, report that having regular sex extends your life by years.

Q. My husband has warts on his hands. Can I catch them if he touches my nether zone?

There is a risk, but it's a slight one. Hand and genital warts are caused by different strains of the human papillomavirus, or HPV. (There are more than 100 strains, and most are actually harmless.) But on rare occasions, the strain of HPV that causes warts like the ones on your husband's hands can indeed lead to warts elsewhere. To be safe, ask your man to wear thin latex gloves during any "play" until his warts are gone. (He can treat them with over-the-counter salicylic acid medication or see a dermatologist for an even faster cure.) Even after his warts are gone, make sure you don't have any cuts, nicks, or open sores down there—these can spread HPV even when all warts have cleared up. Incidentally, the HPV vaccine is no help in this case: It protects against separate strains of HPV that can cause cervical cancer.

· · · · · ·

Q. Can head lice migrate to down below?

No, it's almost as if there's an invisible boundary of sorts on your body. Head lice can get into the hair on your head—all of it: scalp, eyebrows, eyelashes, facial hair. But they won't go any farther south. Pubic lice (you know—"crabs") can migrate north to your armpits and even your eyelashes, but not your scalp. Despite what we'd like to think, head lice are extremely common, especially among children. But pubic lice are a totally different bug; they're considered an STD because they're transmitted through genital-to-genital contact. You can treat both with over-the-counter products.

3 years!
That's how many years regular sex adds to your life.
Source: Mehmet Oz, MD, in *Health* Magazine

Q. I have an itchy bump in my pubic area—how can I tell if it's a bite or an STD?

It could be a herpes outbreak, but if it doesn't develop into a painful or itchy blister within a few days, it's probably not. Herpes blisters also tend to show up in clusters, not as isolated spots. If you're worried, though, make an appointment with your gyno to get it checked out, and avoid sex in the meantime.

The spot could also be one of several minor things—from a pimple (uncommon but not unheard of) to a type of painless cyst called Bartholin's gland cyst, which sometimes shows up on the vagina. If you suspect a cyst, it's nothing to worry about but do have it drained by a doctor. Don't poke at it yourself because it could get infected. Another culprit could be an obstructed hair follicle, which is sometimes caused by shaving. Washing the area carefully and drying it well should help free the impacted hair, but if you begin to see signs of infection (the spot widens or develops a white tip), see your doctor or dermatologist to have the hair removed.

• • • • • • •

Q. Why do I get a headache *after* sex? Am I allergic to my orgasm?

The root cause of your headache—called a "coital headache"—probably isn't your orgasm but the sex itself. Your body is reacting to the fact that sex is a strenuous activity. Or it could be from the increased muscle activity and dilation of blood vessels around your neck and brain as a result of the sex.

I would suggest taking an OTC anti-inflammatory like ibuprofen or a doctor-prescribed migraine med 30 minutes before hitting the sheets. If these headaches get persistently worse or if you start having them at other times, bring them up to your physician. She might want to check for possible medicine complications or even run a few tests to rule out other problems.

NOT TO WORRY!

Meredith and McDreamy may seem to do the deed multiple times a day, but the average American couple has sex one to two times a week, according to University of Chicago research.

73

Q. Can I get HIV from oral sex?

Yes. Although the risk is less than with anal or vaginal sex, there have been cases of transmission through oral sex. Infected blood from the mouth can enter your body through the lining of the vagina. You can also get HIV by performing oral sex because semen or pre-seminal fluid (the little bit of juice on the penis tip) contains the virus. Your risk goes up if you have any sores or cuts in your mouth or vagina (which you may have without even realizing it) and if he ejaculates in your mouth. So it's best to use condoms or dental dams or make sure your partner gets tested before you engage in this kind of intimate behavior.

Q. Is it dangerous to "play" with food during sex? Anything safe to put in my vagina?

The honest truth? It's best not to put anything up there. Vaginal bacteria love to feed on sugar, so foods with a high-sugar content (chocolate sauce, sweet whipped cream, honey, fruit...all the traditional sex-play staples) are a no-no. If anything remains post-sex or isn't washed away quickly, the bacteria, loving their new source of nutrient, will start eating and multiplying and might cause an overgrowth of bacteria, leading to infection. In addition, the sugar can throw off the pH of your vagina, increasing your chances of a yeast infection. Another avoid-at-all-costs: oily foods. They can trap bacteria and are hard to wash off (yuck).

If you really want to mix food and fooling around, just feed each other sexy foods like chocolate-covered strawberries before getting down to business.

65% of women say they don't need to have an orgasm to have satisfying sex.

Source: Health.com poll

Q. This is mortifying, but I've never had an orgasm. Are some people just incapable?

It's extremely rare for a woman to be physically unable to achieve orgasm, though it's not unusual for a woman to think that she's missing the orgasm gene. But unless you've just recently gone from being able to orgasm to not—or you suspect something is interfering with your ability to climax, such as pain during sex or medicines lowering your drive—there's probably no *physical* reason you can't orgasm. Instead, try a few things before giving up on sexual bliss.

First—and this is the hardest part—try to stop focusing on it so much. In women, orgasms are usually as much mental as physical. Unfortunately, that means the more you obsess about it, the less likely you are to get there. Unlike men who—let's be honest—usually have orgasms effortlessly starting in adolescence, many women pass through their 20s, 30s, even beyond without ever experiencing the Big O.

Why is that? While we see women in movies who peak with vaginal sex, in real life, it's just not always that way. The vagina isn't very sensitive to stimulation; the clitoris, which is our version of the penis, needs to be stimulated for orgasm, and the more direct the stimulation the better. (With vaginal sex, you're indirectly stimulating the clitoris at best.) So ask your man for oral sex or manual stimulation of the clitoris: Even if it doesn't send you over the edge, it should feel amazing, which is really the point, right?

Better yet, figure out how to flip your switch on your own. Sometimes this kind of low-pressure practice makes all the difference. Getting hands on with your body is a great way to figure out what you love and what you don't. Then sign your guy up for a tutorial. Chances are he'll love knowing what gets you off.

Q. Lately I'm sore and itchy after sex—could I be allergic to condoms?

It's possible but not all that likely. Latex is in tons of things besides condoms (Band-Aids, dishwashing gloves, balloons, sanitary pads) so if you were allergic to latex, you'd probably know already. What is more likely is you're allergic to another part of the condom—the spermicide or the lubricant. Try a different brand of condom or use one without a lubricant and supply your own, preferably a water-based one because they're way less irritating. That soreness and itchiness could also be a sign of an early-stage yeast infection or bacterial vaginosis (a bacterial infection of the vagina). These are usually also accompanied by discharge, so if your symptoms progress, see your gyno. She'll prescribe either an antifungal medication or antibiotic to help clear it up.

Oh, and is this a new relationship? If so, and you ever have sex without a condom, it's also possible you're allergic to his semen. While it's extremely rare, it happens. And it's a tough problem to solve. Some doctors try slowly increasing your exposure to the semen in hopes you'll no longer have a reaction. But this is tricky and needs to be done and supervised by a doctor.

Q. But wouldn't I know by now if I were allergic to semen?

Surprisingly, you might not. This allergy is usually a reaction to a specific protein in a specific man's semen. So it's completely possible that you wouldn't have had a problem with other guys but just happen to react to your current man.

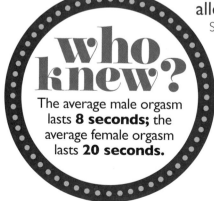

who knew?

The average male orgasm lasts **8 seconds;** the average female orgasm lasts **20 seconds.**

The Frisky 4

Want to feel even more up for action?
Eat these libido-boosting foods.

 ALMONDS: These heart-healthy nuts are rich in zinc, a mineral that boosts libido.

 SEAFOOD: Oysters and other kinds of seafood also serve up zinc. And fish with omega-3 fatty acids like salmon keep your blood pumping and your heart primed for romps.

 DARK CHOCOLATE: Some research shows it ups feel-good chemicals in your brain, putting you in the mood for you-know-what.

 ASPARAGUS: This veggie serves up a hit of vitamin E, helping your body pump out testosterone.

Getting Gorgeous

chapter

5

Stray hairs, weird smells, tattoo regret, oh my!

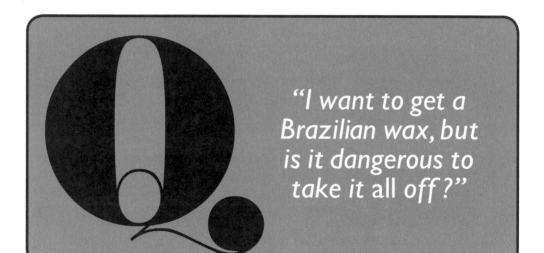

"I want to get a Brazilian wax, but is it dangerous to take it all off?"

Pubic hair prevents chafing of the delicate skin around your vagina when your guy is rubbing against you during sex. Think of it as a buffer from the friction. So if you go completely bare, you may get irritated from sex. Plus, if the waxing causes tiny abrasions in the skin, you are more susceptible to STDs.

Of course, with any bikini wax there is a risk of a bacterial infection. So it's important to make sure the place is licensed and clean. Watch closely to make sure they never wax in the same spot twice (this will up your chance of irritation) or double-dip the wax stick (which can transfer bacteria).

Q. What's up with those UV-light dryers at the nail salon? Could they make you wrinkle faster? Or even give you skin cancer?

Those UV-light dryers are like tiny tanning beds, so you're right to be concerned. While this danger hasn't been looked at in any large-scale studies, dermatologists report finding more skin cancer on the fingers (typically a very rare location) of patients who have frequent exposure to these nail-drying lights. In fact, a recent report in *Archives of Dermatology* said that using them may be a risk factor for the development of skin cancer. Also, we know that UV light increases your risk of cancer (and wrinkles), and if you're going to the nail salon every two weeks (or weekly), that will add up to significant exposure. My two cents? Use them sparingly, or, better yet, let your nails dry on their own. It may take a bit longer, but it's worth the effort to save your skin.

• • • • • • •

Q. I don't have a problem sleeping, so why do I have such dark circles?

A few culprits may have you reaching for the under-eye concealer. Sinus blockage triggered by a food or seasonal allergy can cause swelling of the tiny blood vessels near the surface of the skin, giving you "darkened" areas around your nose and eyes. An allergist can determine an allergy trigger, but if yours is seasonal or the irritant is unavoidable, an OTC drug like Claritin or Zyrtec should help.

How's your diet? A vitamin deficiency may also cause circles. Take a daily multi if you don't already, and add a night cream or facial mask containing vitamins K and A (aka retinol) to your regimen.

30% of women have tried giving themselves a bikini wax.

Source: Health.com poll

Of course, your genes may also be to blame. Some women have a genetic predisposition to excessive pigmentation in the area. Laser surgery—which resurfaces the skin and destroys the highly pigmented cells—is a solution, but it doesn't come cheap (it costs thousands of dollars) or easy (expect a lengthy recovery period). Cosmetic-filler injections like Juvéderm or Restylane are a popular alternative (they fill in the sunken areas that cause shadowing), again for a pretty penny— $500 to $800 per treatment, which lasts only about six months.

But before you break the bank, try simply squeezing in even a half-hour extra of sleep because fatigue can dull your skin and make any discoloration more visible. Even if you don't have a sleep problem per se, your body may just need a little more rest than you're currently giving it.

> **PSST, FROM DR. RAJ!**
> *Bring a list of everything you're taking—including prescriptions, over-the-counter medicines, vitamins, and herbal remedies—to your doctor visit. This will ensure we don't prescribe something that'll react with your other treatments.*

Q. I just found a—gasp!—gray pubic hair. If I remove it, will a thousand more grow back?

A thousand? No. One? Yes. We think we see more gray hairs after we pluck one because gray hairs tend to occur in patches.

Just like gray hairs on your head, gray pubic hairs come from hair follicles that have lost their pigment (melanin). A new hair that grows from the same follicle will also be gray. So go ahead and pluck it if you want, but know it'll be back.

• • • • • •

Q. Is it true there's lead in my red lipstick?

This is one Internet rumor that's true: Some red lipsticks do contain lead. In fact, a few independent studies by the Food and Drug Administration and the Campaign for Safe Cosmetics have found low levels of lead in many red tubes, and not just the cheap ones. Some really expensive brands pack more lead than drugstore lipsticks.

What's the harm in lead? While this toxic metal is far more dangerous to children (another reason you may not want a lead-loaded tube in your handbag), it can harm adults, too, building up in our bodies over time and causing high blood pressure and anemia, as well as reproductive and neurological problems. But don't panic—there hasn't been a single reported case of lead poisoning from lip color.

Still, why chance it? Although the levels are low (less than you get from drinking tap water in many areas of the country), if you reapply your "poppy red" several times a day, it could build up in your body. So it makes sense to check www.safecosmetics.org and see if your favorite brand is safe.

HOW **BAD** IS IT *REALLY?*
To use cotton swabs to dig out my earwax

Not a good idea. Earwax, while kind of gross, is actually a good thing: It's a sticky shield that protects your eardrum from bacteria and dirt. Typically, old wax dries up and falls out or washes away, but sometimes it builds up and causes pain or hearing problems. Some of us are just waxier than others (don't worry; it's not a sign of illness). Don't try to go in deep using cotton swabs or anything else: You risk perforating your eardrum or pushing water or dirt deep in the ear, which can cause infection. Use swabs only on the outer part of the inner ear, and wipe away visible wax with a warm, damp washcloth. If wax buildup muffles your hearing or causes pain, see your doctor. She may prescribe eardrops or recommend an OTC product. She can also remove buildup with a bulb syringe. But don't try this at home!

5: Getting Gorgeous

Q. Please tell me there's something I can do about my hairy butt.

If you're talking about the hair between the anus and vagina, that's a tough spot—and a tender one, too. Hair-removal creams are off limits because they can cause severe irritation to your delicate skin. I also wouldn't recommend putting a razor to the area because of the risk of infection.

Waxing at least some of the easy-to-reach hairs is an option, but it's not going to be a fun visit. It's a very sensitive area (did I mention that?!); take ibuprofen a half-hour before you go.

If this hair really bothers you—and I don't think it should because it's totally normal—laser hair removal may be worth considering. Yes, it's expensive, and, yes, it requires several visits, but it's a safe (as long as you go to a board-certified dermatologist) and fairly permanent solution.

• • • • • •

Q. I got a little drunk last weekend and ended up with a tattoo. Now I'm worried that I caught something serious like hepatitis. Should I panic?

Not yet. Your risk of exposure is very low—as long as the tattoo parlor was sanitary and used needles that were properly sterilized.

If you remember where the tattoo parlor was (check your purse for a receipt), go back and make sure they're licensed. (Whenever you get inked, make sure to go to a licensed tattoo parlor.) If they are, they're probably sterilizing their equipment. If the place is "sketchy" or can't produce a license, you have more to worry about.

In any case, to ease your mind and protect your health, it's a good idea to have your doctor test you for possible infections. You'll need to be tested twice—once as soon as possible and once in a few weeks because some viruses take several weeks to show up.

In the unlikely case that something turns up, your doc will walk you through what to do next. Chances are you should be fine, but it is best to be sure.

Decode Your Beauty Problems

1) CRACKED LIPS

What it may mean: A vitamin deficiency, which can cause cracking at the corners of your mouth.

Solution: Have your doc check your levels, and be sure to take a multivitamin.

2) WHITE LINES ON YOUR NAIL

What it may mean: You likely injured your nail bed without even realizing it.

Solution: Once the nail grows long enough, simply cut the damaged part off.

3) BRIGHT PINK GUMS

What it may mean: You grind your teeth. Clenching puts pressure on gums, causing them to redden.

Solution: Ask your doctor for a mouth guard, which prevents damage from middle-of-the-night grinding.

4) DARK CIRCLES UNDER YOUR EYES

What it may mean: You have allergies, which can cause congestion of the blood vessels in that area.

Solution: Try an over-the-counter non-sedating allergy medication daily. Also try to get more rest because fatigue makes this problem worse.

Q. Why would I suddenly start getting facial hair?

As we get older, it's normal to get more facial hair, which is darker and coarser than those fine hairs many of us have when we're younger. But if this change is sudden and dramatic, there is probably a hormonal imbalance going on (more androgens, which are male hormones, than estrogen). You should visit your doc to be checked for hormone changes that could be related to menopause, medicines (e.g. steroids, oral contraceptives), polycystic ovarian syndrome, or, in rare cases, a hormone-secreting tumor.

Assuming there's nothing major going on, you may just be genetically predisposed to having facial hair (thanks, Grandma!). But no need to live with it. Here's a quickie guide to how you can deal with unwanted hair:

Pluck away: It's cheap, it's DIY…but it's a lot of work, depending on how many hairs you have and how quickly they grow back. If you go this route, invest in a good sturdy pair of slanted-tip tweezers and a magnifying mirror.
Bleach them: If it's just the darkness of that hair you can't stand, try a bleaching cream. Caveat: Avoid this method if you have very sensitive skin.
Remove 'em at home: Depilatory creams—which work by dissolving the hair at the base of the follicle—are cheap and easy to buy at the drugstore, but they can be irritating. Other cons: They typically don't remove all the hair, and the results last only one to two weeks.
Wax 'em off: Find a good aesthetician, and book a standing waxing appointment every few weeks.
Laser 'em off: After three treatments, you should notice a 50 to 70 percent decrease in those pesky dark hairs. The downside, of course, is the price: A single laser treatment can run as much as $350. To find a qualified doc in your area, ask your derm if she does it or, if not, if she can recommend a colleague. Don't trust your face to anyone but a board-certified dermatologist who owns her own equipment and does laser treatments regularly.
Slow their growth: You can also ask your doc about Vaniqa, a prescription drug that slows facial-hair growth.

70% of women have shared lip gloss or mascara with a friend.

Source: Health.com poll

Q. The rose tattoo on my left breast used to seem so cute, but now that my boobs have started to sag, it looks scary. How can I get rid of it?

I'll give it to you straight: It's a lot easier to get a tattoo than to get rid of one (which is why I urge women to think twice about getting inked in the first place). Why? With tattoos, ink is inserted deep into the dermal layer of your skin, so total removal is often impossible. But, thanks to the magic of lasers, you can now erase most of it—or at least lighten it—without that much scarring.

This is good news because tattoo removal used to involve lots of procedures and scarring, without great results. Now the process is done with lasers and is far more effective: The ink takes in the laser energy and is broken up into tiny particles that are then absorbed by your body.

It's not foolproof, though, depending on what kind of ink was used (and how long ago you got your tat). Also, certain colors such as yellow and green are tougher to remove. More caveats: It's painful (lasers inflame the skin) and expensive (as much as $350 a session), and you may need multiple follow-up treatments (depending on the size of your flower and the types of ink used). Also, there is a risk of hypo- or hyperpigmentation, meaning the site might be lighter or darker than the surrounding skin after the tattoo is removed.

Still want it gone? Talk to your dermatologist to see if she does the procedure or can recommend someone who does.

HOW **BAD** IS IT *REALLY?*

To borrow a friend's razor

Bad. Razors can pick up traces of blood and other bodily secretions, so you are essentially exposing yourself to your friend's blood and any infections or STDs lurking in her body (hepatitis B or C, herpes, HIV, etc.). And many women have these infections without realizing it, so you likely wouldn't know your friend's status. My feeling? Don't chance it.

5: Getting Gorgeous

Q. I heard that dark hair dye causes cancer, and I'm worried. Does that mean I should go blonde?

No need to. Before the early 1970s, many hair dyes contained buckets of chemicals, some of which were shown to cause cancer in animals. The darker dyes contained more potential carcinogens (cancer-causing agents), so they were believed to be riskier. Since then, dye manufacturers have removed many—though not all—of these toxic chemicals.

The studies that have turned up a link between dye and cancer have looked at people who used the older, more toxic formulas. One reported an increased risk of bladder cancer in male hairdressers and barbers (who had been exposed to these old-school chemicals on a daily basis for many years). Another study found that women who used hair dye frequently prior to 1980 had an increased risk of non-Hodgkin lymphoma, but those who colored their hair frequently after 1980 did not have any increased risk. Since there's no good recent research showing a connection between hair color and cancer, most experts say not to worry.

Still, it makes sense to limit your exposure to these chemicals. Use gloves when applying the dye. If you're pregnant, many obstetricians will recommend you not dye your hair during the first trimester (while baby is undergoing major neurological development), but they say that it's probably safe to do so in the last two trimesters. Limit the time dye is on your head, and wash your scalp well after removing it. Also, consider waiting until your hair is turning gray, rather than going auburn or jet black just because you're looking for a change, to cut your long-term exposure to the chemicals. You can also switch to a temporary dye, which is less toxic, or henna, which is usually all natural.

6 Surprising Hair-Loss Culprits

Notice thinning? Talk to your doctor about whether one of the following could be to blame.

1) A SCREWY THYROID. An overactive or underactive thyroid (diagnosed with a blood test) can cause hair loss on your head and elsewhere.

2) POST-PREGNANCY HORMONAL FLUCTUATIONS. You shed more hair after giving birth (after shedding less during pregnancy). It all evens out after six months or so.

3) YOUR HAIRCARE REGIMEN. Excessive blow-drying and hot-ironing, chemicals from dye and chemical straightening, and even too-tight ponytails can cause hair to break and thin out. Go easy to reverse this problem.

4) THAT CRASH DIET. Lack of protein and iron in your diet can wreak havoc with hair—try eating a little extra lean red meat and hard-boiled eggs.

5) MEDS. Some antidepressants, anti-arthritis drugs, and even birth control pills can cause thinning. Ask your MD if you can switch to a drug that doesn't have this side effect.

6) YOUR GENES. You may have a common hereditary condition: alopecia. If so, your doc can prescribe Women's Rogaine, the only FDA-approved treatment for hereditary hair loss in women.

Q. Egad, why are my eyelashes falling out?

Believe it or not, it could be your beauty routine. Are you tugging on them too hard when you use an eyelash curler? Also consider your mascara: Are you using one that's harsh on your eyes or hard to remove (big culprit: waterproof mascaras)? You may even be allergic to that wand, triggering lash loss. Switch to a hypoallergenic mascara (get one that's especially for sensitive eyes) and a gentle eye-makeup remover and see if your problem gets better.

If switching up your products doesn't help, a hormonal issue like hypo-thyroidism might be to blame. Your doctor can run a blood test to look at hormone levels. Medications (such as steroids) and an autoimmune disorder called alopecia areata are other possibilities, so do talk to your doc.

* * * * * *

Q. My toenails are so yellow and bumpy that I'm too embarrassed to get a pedicure. Do I have a fungus or something?

Sure sounds like it. You probably picked it up at the gym. I'd hold off on a pedicure, not because it's embarrassing but because it's risky. If you get a cut or scratch during a pedicure, the infection could spread to your blood-stream. An unsightly toenail or two pales in comparison to an infection in your bloodstream.

You can attack the fungus with prescription meds like Lamisil or Sporanox, but know that these meds are expensive, must be taken for at least three months, and in some cases don't do the trick. So some people choose to simply put up with fungus. Unfortunately, home remedies—such as soaking your feet in Listerine or Vicks VapoRub—typically don't work.

To avoid picking up nail fungus in the first place (or spreading it around), be sure to wear flip-flops in the shower and locker room at the gym. And if your man has toenail fungus, wear socks to bed to keep your feet from touching his during the night, and don't share toenail clippers.

5 Signs That Spa Isn't Safe

 NO LICENSE. If a license isn't prominently displayed or if they aren't able or willing to produce one, you should go somewhere else.

 IFFY FOOT BATHS. Make sure the pedicure tubs are fully drained and scrubbed after every use. If you don't see someone scrubbing, slip on your shoes and run. Warm water is an ideal breeding ground for bacteria and fungus.

 SCARY BATHROOMS. Rest rooms are a good indication of the priority a salon places on cleanliness. If the ladies room is a mess or reeks, you can assume they're not big on cleaning.

 BARELY SANITIZED TOOLS. If they aren't fully submerged in disinfecting liquid, they're still dirty.

 STRONG OR FUNNY ODORS. If that spa or salon reeks of nail polish fumes, other chemicals, or even aromatherapy products, the spa isn't well ventilated. Strong fumes can give you a headache and respiratory problems.

Q. I use deodorant every day, but my pits still reek. What should I do?

Smelly pits are the pits, but they're usually treatable. First, think about what you've been eating or drinking lately: Alcohol, garlic, onions, and spicy foods all contain chemicals that get secreted through your pores, upping your odor. If you've been on a Mexican or Indian food bender, try cutting back and see if that helps your problem.

Wearing clothing made from breathable fabrics like cotton—that wick moisture away from your pits—may also help; where there's moisture, there's greater likelihood of bacterial growth, which can cause a stench. It's also worth trying a stronger antiperspirant-deodorant, such as an unscented men's product or any with at least 12 percent aluminum chloride. Apply it before bed and again as soon as you get out of the shower in the morning.

If the extreme odor persists, see your doctor to rule out a thyroid problem or hormonal changes related to your menstrual cycle or menopause. She may recommend hormone therapy or a prescription-strength antiperspirant-deodorant, which contains 20 percent aluminum chloride.

PSST, FROM DR. RAJ!
Don't shave your legs the day of your pedicure because even a small cut can be an entry point for tiny bacteria and other infection-causing bugs.

Q. I know lots of women get bikini waxes, but I prefer to go au naturel. Any harm in leaving all that hair?

None at all. Pubic hair protects your delicate vaginal and genital skin from chafing (due to sex or even your under-wear). And by not waxing or shaving, you're avoiding the risk of infections, burns, or tiny cuts that up your risk of contracting an STD. So, by all means, keep your down-there hair.

• • • • • •

Q. My feet are cracked and coated with white scum. Do I need a pedicure—or a trip to the doc?

Actually, neither. Cracked heels are a very common problem and usually fixable at home.

Dry skin is the problem. Skin dries out when we wear shoes without socks, and you get chafing between your heels and shoes. For many women, it's just a cosmetic issue—unsightly sure, but not painful. However, the cracks in the skin can become so deep that they are painful to stand on, and they can bleed or become infected in the most severe cases.

Hold off on getting a pedicure until you've got the dryness under control a bit more. Though unlikely, there may be tiny abrasions in the skin, and if any bacteria were to get in, unsightly feet might be the least of your problems. Instead, use a pumice stone or heel file to remove the rough, calloused skin. Each time you shower, gently scrub for 30 to 45 seconds on each heel. You won't remove it all at once, but over time, you'll see a change. Then moisturize with a thick lotion—preferably one that has cocoa butter or tea tree oil. At night, it's a good idea to apply a thick layer of lotion and then slide on some socks—this helps keep the moisturizer from wiping off on your sheets so it can penetrate while you sleep.

If the cracks become worse or the heels don't improve after treating, see your dermatologist. She may need to prescribe an antifungal cream.

Q. What is this gunk in my belly button, and why does it smell so bad?

Since you asked: It's a mixture of lint, dirt, dried sweat, and dead skin cells. If you have an innie (and 90 percent of us do), the belly button is an area that can trap moisture and bacteria (which love moist environments). It starts to smell when bacteria eat sweat and release an odor.

To stop the stench: First, clean the area well during showers, and be sure to dry it. If you're going to be extra sweaty (like during workouts or in the summer's heat), sprinkle some baby powder or cornstarch in there. Also, a tiny bit of deodorant on a cotton swab rubbed gently into the belly button may help.

If the smell is really strong (as in: other people notice it), see your doctor. You may actually have a fungal or bacterial infection and need medication.

· · · · · ·

Q. After years of clear skin, I've got zits again. Is it something I'm eating?

Probably not. There's absolutely no research to support the old urban legend that foods like chocolate or pizza cause acne. Instead, the culprit could be lurking in your cosmetic case, bathroom, or laundry room. Makeup, soaps, shampoos, or even laundry detergents can cause an allergic reaction that causes breakouts. If you've recently switched brands, go back to your old ones and see if that helps.

If your acne persists, see a dermatologist. She can figure out if your pimples are actually due to rosacea—a common skin condition that can cause acne and redness—or hormonal fluctuations brought on by your menstrual cycle or menopause. They're treatable, so it's worth a doctor's visit.

Decode Your Moles

How can you tell a mole that's normal from one that's not? Here are the 5 danger signs:

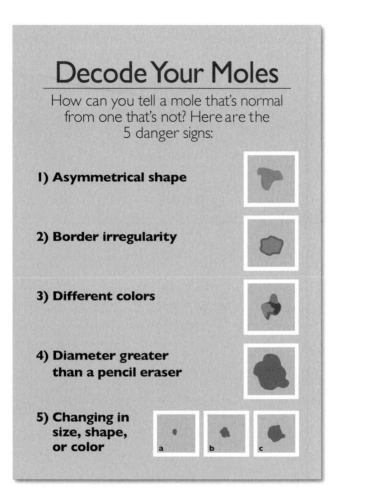

1) **Asymmetrical shape**

2) **Border irregularity**

3) **Different colors**

4) **Diameter greater than a pencil eraser**

5) **Changing in size, shape, or color**

a   b   c

In the Stirrups

chapter 6

*All the burning
questions you're dying
to ask your gyno
(but won't)*

6: In the Stirrups

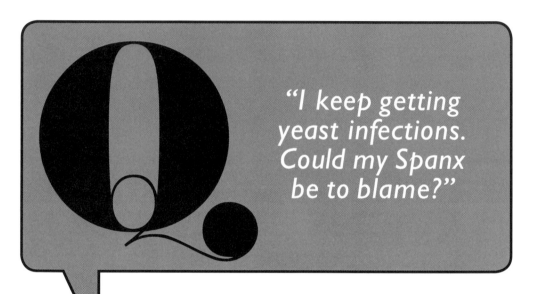

Q. "I keep getting yeast infections. Could my Spanx be to blame?"

a Much as I hate to say anything bad about my beloved Spanx, the body shapers could be contributing to your problem. We all have some vaginal yeast, but when that yeast multiplies, it becomes a problem. What makes it spread like crazy? A warm, damp crotch, for one. So when you wear underwear or body-shaping apparel like Spanx that is tight and made of a non-breathable synthetic fabric, you're setting the stage for overgrowth.

Spanx are hard to quit, for sure. You don't have to go cold turkey. Just save your slimmers for short-term use and special occasions, rather than using them as your go-to everyday undergarment.

Q. Can my gyno tell if I had sex last night?

Hmm, that depends. If she's just feeling around in there (as she would during a regular pelvic exam), then no, because normal vaginal secretions won't feel any different if there is sperm or semen mixed in. But if your doc examines your discharge under a microscope (which she may if you have symptoms of an infection), she may spot sperm since they can survive for a couple of days inside your body.

If you know you're having a pap smear, though, try to skip sex for 48 hours prior to the appointment, because the test's accuracy could be affected by the sperm, lube, or even the act of intercourse itself (it can damage the cells on the cervix).

· · · · · · ·

Q. If men are hardwired to be visual, how could male ob/gyns not occasionally get aroused on the job?

Have you ever heard the phrase, "Familiarity breeds contempt"? Well male gynos see, on a daily basis, so many vaginas, breasts, etc—in all sorts of shapes, sizes, and not-so-pretty conditions—that the last thing they are thinking about is sex. They're in medical mode, thinking about discharges, conditions, and leaks as they focus on you and your health.

That said, there are exceptions to every rule, and if you are getting some creepy vibes when you see your doctor (of either sex), it's time to switch. And remember, there should be a female medical assistant or nurse in the room whenever you are being examined by a male gyno. Being without one is to his disadvantage, too. Examining you alone opens him up to lawsuits: Any woman can say she was touched inappropriately, and there would be no witness to back up the doctor. So if you're in for an exam and he doesn't call in an assistant, ask for one—even if it is momentarily awkward.

75% of women will have at least one vaginal yeast infection during their lives.

Source: Mayo Clinic

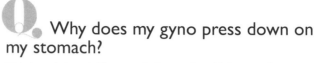

Q. Why does my gyno press down on my stomach?

This is an integral (if not entirely comfortable) part of your exam. She's feeling the size, shape, and mobility of your uterus, and checking for the presence of any cysts, fibroids, or tumors of your ovaries, uterus, or fallopian tubes. Since many of these organs are deep inside the abdomen, she may have to press hard, but it is an important part of the exam.

Your gyno might also insert two fingers into your vagina at the same time as she is pressing on your lower abdomen. This is called the bimanual exam, and she's checking for any tenderness in your internal organs. It will be a little uncomfortable, so expect some minor pain. However, if it's more than a little painful, let her know. She might want to feel around more or run tests to see if there's something causing you to yowl.

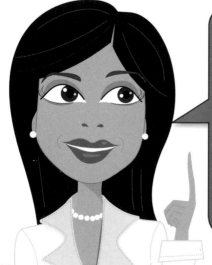

PSST, FROM DR. RAJ!
Wondering what your gyno is up to down there? Go ahead and ask. You'll feel less anxious if you understand exactly what your doctor is checking. And talking throughout the exam will prevent you from holding your breath, which helps cut the pain level of the exam.

Q. How many C-sections can I have without my uterus flat-out giving out? I had one baby by C but want to have a big family.

With every C-section you have, your chance of serious complications—such as uterine rupture, placenta abnormalities, and postpartum hemorrhage—go up. These problems can be very dangerous for you and your baby. But it's hard to give a simple answer to this question: Every woman heals differently, and while one woman may be able to have three C-sections safely, another may be advised to stop after just one Cesarean because of significant scar tissue or poor healing.

But even one Cesarean section carries some risk. Your abdomen and uterus are being cut in order to remove your baby. And as with any surgery, there is the chance of bleeding, damage to other organs, blood clots, scar tissue, and adhesions. Subsequent C's are riskier than the first one, so the decision to have an initial one shouldn't be taken lightly. I've heard of women (even some physicians) who schedule a C-section for a first baby for the sake of convenience. This is major surgery, people! So unless it's medically necessary, you should take the vaginal route.

My advice: Discuss your big-family dreams with your doctor as soon as possible. She knows you best, and can give an answer that's based on your individual health history. There's recent evidence suggesting that some women can safely have a vaginal birth after Cesarean (VBAC). Ask your OB for her views on VBAC, and whether it could be a safe plan for babies number two, three, and four.

TRUE OR FALSE?

Yeast infections are a sign of HIV.

False. Yeast infections are so incredibly common in women, I would hardly call them—even if they're recurring—a sign of HIV. Still, if you have more than three battles with yeast in a six-month period, consider it a sign to talk to your doc.

It is true that people who have a compromised immune system for any reason (and yes, HIV is one of them, along with cancer, diabetes, steroid use, and chronic illness) are more prone to getting yeast infections. Bottom line: If you get yeast infections often, don't panic, but consider it a sign to talk to your doc.

6: In the Stirrups

Q. During my annual checkup, my gyno feels around inside me—what's she groping for in there?

She's feeling around for any abnormal lumps or bumps on your labia, your cervix (the opening to your uterus), and the lips of your vagina, as well as inside your vagina. She's also checking for tenderness of the cervix—which could be a sign of inflammation due to an STD or a cyst on your ovaries. In addition, she's feeling for any abnormalities of the uterus. These are all things you might not feel, but are important to pick up early. It may be uncomfortable, but shouldn't be painful. If it is, by all means speak up.

· · · · · · ·

Q. How many days can you forget to take the Pill without getting pregnant?

None. Skipping even one day can increase your chance of getting pregnant. One quick exception: If you skipped taking one of the placebo pills at the end of your cycle, you're probably okay. In reality, we don't even have to take those pills; they're usually just sugar pills and contain no hormones. Their sole purpose is to keep you in the habit of taking a pill every day, reducing your chances of missing a pill.

If you realize you've spaced out on one dose, quickly take it or just double up (take two pills) the next day. But if you've missed more than one pill, don't try to catch up; call your doctor. And in either case, use another form of birth control (condoms, for example) for that entire cycle, just to be safe.

Get B6 to Beat Bloat

Vitamin B6 acts as a mild diuretic, making you pee more. (It may also help your mood: B6 deficiency has been linked with depression.) That's a good thing when you're retaining water before your period, thanks to high levels of estrogen. The NIH recommends you get 1.3 milligrams of the vitamin every day. Eat these to get your B6:

 BAKED POTATO is one of the best natural sources of B6: A medium potato has 0.74 mg.

 BREAKFAST CEREAL that's fortified (like bran flakes with raisins) has 1.0 mg per serving.

 BEEF Three ounces serves up about 0.4 mg.

 BANANA contains 0.43 mg.

P.S. You can also take a B6 supplement, but not one with more than 50 milligrams a day. Higher levels may cause nerve damage.

Q. My gyno told me I have a tipped uterus. Is that bad? Will I have trouble getting pregnant?

You won't have any problems getting pregnant—at least not from your tipped uterus. A tipped uterus just means that rather than the usual straight vertical position the uterus normally sits in, yours is tilted toward the back. It's so common—about one in five women has it—that it's considered a "normal variant."

I'd guess most women don't know they have this variant until their gyno does a pelvic exam. While some women with a tipped uterus experience pain with intercourse or with their periods, most women don't have any symptoms at all.

There are a few conditions that may cause a tipped uterus (such as endometriosis or pelvic inflammatory disease) and affect your fertility. So if you're having a hard time conceiving, and your gyno just noticed your tipped uterus, it's worth having a conversation with her to see if there's any connection between your uterus's position and your fertility challenges.

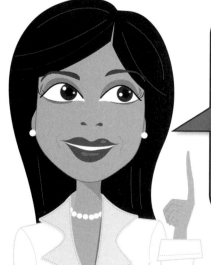

PSST, FROM DR. RAJ!
Ask for the smallest speculum for your body size. A 28-year-old who hasn't had a child won't need the same speculum as a 50-year-old with five kids. A right-sized tool will make your cervical exam much more comfortable.

Q. My doc thinks I have uterine fibroids. What are they?

Fibroids are incredibly common (as many as three out of four women have them) non-cancerous uterine growths. Most women don't know they even have fibroids. But some notice heavy menstrual bleeding, prolonged periods (more than seven days), pelvic pressure or pain, frequent urination, and, very rarely, infertility.

Q. So how did I get them?

We don't know the cause of uterine fibroids, but suspects include hormones (estrogen and progesterone stimulate development of the uterine lining), genetic mutations in uterine cells (fibroids contain alterations in genes), or bodily chemicals (such as insulin-like growth factor, which normally helps the body maintain healthy tissue).

Q. So what should I do about them?

If you have no symptoms, the best thing is to wait and monitor the fibroids. If you do notice heavy periods, pelvic pain, or one of the other signs, your doctor will likely run blood tests and check your uterus with a sonogram.

If you do have fibroids, you may be put on a med that targets the hormones (estrogen and progesterone) that regulate your menstrual cycle. Even if your fibroids aren't caused by hormones, this medication will help. While they don't eliminate fibroids, they may shrink them.

who knew?

We're born with all the eggs we'll ever have (unlike men, who produce new sperm daily throughout most of their lives).

6: In the Stirrups

YOUR DOCTOR MAY SUGGEST ONE OF THESE PROCEDURES FOR FIBROIDS:

• **Uterine artery embolization** is a minimally invasive procedure that cuts off the blood flow to the fibroids, starving them so they die. Downside: It doesn't prevent new fibroids from forming.

• **Myolysis** is a laparoscopic procedure that uses a laser to destroy the fibroids and shrink the blood vessels that were supplying them. Cryomyolysis is a similar procedure; it uses liquid nitrogen to freeze the fibroids.

• **Endometrial ablation:** In this procedure, an instrument uses microwave energy or an electric current to destroy the uterine lining. But it isn't an option if you want to have kids. It also doesn't treat fibroids outside the interior of your uterus.

• **Hysterectomy**, or removal of the uterus, is the only guaranteed way to get rid of fibroids. But it's major surgery and not right for someone who still wants children. Because of this, many doctors recommend **myomectomy**, a surgical procedure that removes the fibroids, leaving the uterus in place and able to support a growing fetus. The fibroids may grow back, though.

Q. Hysterectomy? Isn't that operation out of vogue?

You're right, there are plenty of options between doing nothing and removing your uterus altogether. Today most doctors will encourage you to try something else before taking that step. It's major surgery, so if a doctor recommends it, be sure to discuss all the other options.

Decode Your Pelvic Cramps

REGULAR MENSTRUAL CRAMPS

What They Feel Like: Monthly throbbing in your lower abdomen.

Caused By: Uterine contractions during menses that help expel the lining of the uterus.

Rx: These contractions are triggered by chemicals called prostaglandins, so anti-inflammatories like ibuprofen help because they temporarily stop your body from producing them.

ECTOPIC PREGNANCY

What They Feel Like: This cramping may start mild but will likely lead to very severe abdominal pain, often with heavy bleeding. You may also feel pain in your shoulder.

Caused By: An ectopic pregnancy, which means the fertilized egg implants outside the uterus—usually in a fallopian tube.

Rx: Go straight to your doctor or ER since this is an emergency condition. If found very early, a hormone can be injected to stop the egg from developing. If it's not early enough, the developing egg is removed with surgery.

ENDOMETRIOSIS

What They Feel Like: These cramps feel very similar to menstrual cramps, but they can occur at other times—during ovulation and while you're having sex, for instance—and can also cause bleeding at other times of the month.

Caused By: Endometrial tissue gone wild. The endometrial tissue that normally lines just the uterus grows elsewhere in the body, usually within the pelvic region. This misplaced tissue can grow, break down, and bleed monthly—just like the lining of your uterus.

Rx: Treatment is either with hormones (to stop the endometrial implants from spreading), anti-inflammatories, or surgery to remove the endometrial growths altogether.

6: In the Stirrups

Q. **My doctor told me to rinse out my diaphragm with soap and water, but does that *really* sterilize it?**

No need to reach for the antibacterial dishwashing detergent. You're not really trying to sterilize your diaphragm; there's no need to, because it's not going to protect you if your partner has a sexually transmitted disease anyway. You're just trying to clean it post-sex. Use a mild soap and water to gently scrub the diaphragm. Then let it air-dry, and store it in a closed container. Be gentle when you clean it, though; you don't want to cause any tears. And always check for small holes by filling it with water and seeing if there are any leaks. If so, dump it and get a new one.

· · · · · · ·

Q. **My sister says it's OK to wash your vagina with very mild soap in the shower, but I thought soap down there was bad. Who's right?**

You both are. You're right that your vagina actually does a really good job of keeping itself clean, and it doesn't need a lot of help from you. But a gentle cleansing with a mild soap or just warm water is fine for most women, so no harm in what your sister advocates. You just don't want be overzealous about the scrubbing and sudsing, even during your period: That could upset the balance of "good" and "bad" bacteria down there, leaving you with a yeast infection or bacterial vaginosis. Remember to rinse and dry thoroughly.

For a small number of women, some soaps, bubble baths, bath gels and salts, and even scented panty liners can cause itching, redness, or hives. If you're in this camp, avoid products with added fragrance or perfumes (check ingredients carefully). Opt for pH balanced and hypoallergenic soaps, which are less likely to irritate your vagina.

87% of women have held up a mirror to look at themselves down there.

Source: Health.com poll

Q. When I go for my gyno checkup, why do I have to pee in a cup? I hate that part!

I know women with a shy bladder dread this part of the exam, but there is a point—I promise. Your urine can reveal valuable information about what's going on inside you. As weird as it sounds, the first thing your doctor wants to see is how your pee looks. Is it a healthy shade of yellow? Is it cloudy or clear? She'll test it for blood, excess protein, sugar, bacteria, and white blood cells—all possible markers for dehydration, infection, or diseases like diabetes, high blood pressure, or kidney or liver disease. Sometimes, a urine test can diagnose a problem before you have a single symptom, helping you to get prompt treatment.

What the Heck are Ovarian Cysts?

Definition: fluid-filled sacs on or in your ovaries

Cause: Your ovaries grow cyst-like structures called follicles each month. Follicles produce the hormones estrogen and progesterone and release an egg when you ovulate. Sometimes, though, they just keep growing instead of deflating as they normally would, forming a cyst.

Symptoms: An ovarian cyst can be asymptomatic. Other women feel pain or pelvic pressure. If one bursts, you'll often know it: It usually causes sharp, even excruciating pain in the lower abdomen.

Treatment: The majority of ovarian cysts disappear without treatment. If you have a cyst, your doc will monitor it with ultrasounds. If she thinks it's too large or worries that it's something else, she may recommend surgery to remove it.

Reassuring fact: Having ovarian cysts during your childbearing years does not mean you're at increased risk of ovarian cancer.

In Meno Mode

Q. How can I tell if I'm in perimenopause?

Perimenopause—the time before menopause when your ovaries pump out less and less estrogen—varies widely from woman to woman. Some women have symptoms for years and years, while others will only have them for the last few months of perimenopause when estrogen levels decline rapidly. You may notice hot flashes, vaginal dryness, irregular periods, urinary incontinence, decreased interest in sex, breast tenderness, pain with sex, and mood swings (ahh…the joys of being a woman).

The only way to know for sure if you're in perimenopause is to have your doctor check your hormone levels. But you won't know after one blood test. You'll have to have several blood draws over a period of several months to determine if your estrogen levels are heading south. If they are and you're very uncomfortable, talk to your doc about whether hormone replacement is safe for you.

If you notice menopause-like symptoms but blood tests don't show declining estrogen levels, your ob/gyn may want to check for other problems, such as an ovarian cyst.

• • • • • •

Q. Help, I've turned into crazy-mood-swing lady!

Know this: It's not easy to adjust to lower hormone levels. What you're experiencing—while annoying—is completely normal; it's not a sign you're losing your mind. And these emotional ups and downs will settle down once your body adapts.

So what can you do in the meantime? Give yourself permission to slow down, and try some basic relaxation techniques. Sit down and count slowly to 10, as you inhale and exhale. Or close your eyes and visualize a place you find soothing. If you haven't tried yoga or meditation classes before, now is the perfect time to give it a go.

I can tell you that exhaustion makes mood swings way worse, so make it your mission to get an extra half-hour of sleep each night. Cut back on caffeine and get some regular physical activity each day (but not right before bed) to avoid tossing and turning.

Above all, remember that you don't have to suffer, so talk to your doctor. You may want to consider going on antidepressants (which can ease some of the emotional and physical symptoms of menopause), or even hormone-replacement therapy, depending on your health history.

• • • • • •

Q. Is it true men go through meno too?

It's sort of true, but it's not really comparable to our change. Just as our estrogen levels fall as we age, men's testosterone levels decline over the years—a process called andropause. The similarities stop there.

The testosterone levels usually don't decline dramatically (at least not compared to women's estrogen levels), and it's unclear what (if any) effects the decline has on a man. It might affect his energy, muscle mass, bone density, and libido, but it's unclear if it really does. (And many older men—Hugh Hefner comes to mind—still have plenty of libido well into old age). Testosterone replacement isn't recommended unless the levels are very low.

HOW **BAD** IS IT *REALLY?*

To lie to your doc about how much you smoke and drink

It's worse than you think, because it hurts your doc's ability to do her job. Smoking and drinking up your risk for cancer, high blood pressure, blood clots, and strokes, plus heart, liver, and lung diseases. If you want your MD to give you the right diagnosis, you need to share. Other reasons to spill: Alcohol can interfere or react with certain medicines, so if she doesn't know you enjoy a nightly glass or two of wine, she could inadvertently prescribe you something that won't be effective, or even interacts badly with the booze. Just remember, your doctor isn't there to judge; she's there to help you get and stay well.

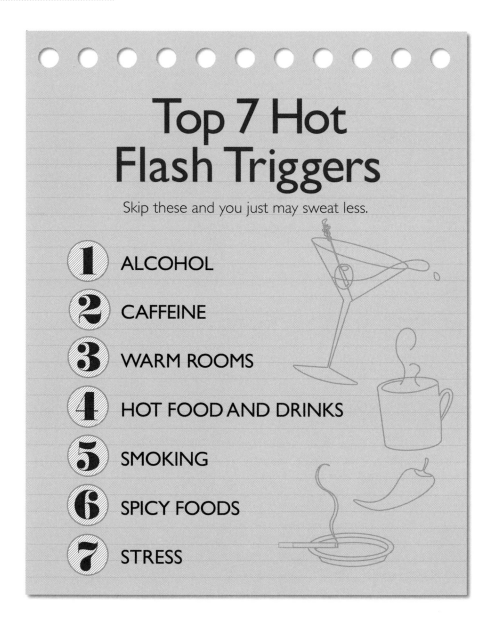

Top 7 Hot Flash Triggers

Skip these and you just may sweat less.

1. ALCOHOL
2. CAFFEINE
3. WARM ROOMS
4. HOT FOOD AND DRINKS
5. SMOKING
6. SPICY FOODS
7. STRESS

Q. Help, I'm having full-on hot flashes during important meetings at work. Please tell me there's something I can do about them!

Three out of four women will have hot flashes during menopause, so take solace, my sweaty sister—you're not alone. These flashes can be mild (you feel like you need to fan yourself with your hand) or severe (a longing to strip down to your bra and panties to relieve the fire).

My advice is the same either way: Keep cool by layering your outfits with breathable, heat-wicking fabrics. This way you can shed a layer (or three) when the hot flashes kick in.

You can also talk to your doctor about prescription medicines. Depending on your individual heart-disease or cancer risk factors, estrogen replacement may be an option for you. If not estrogen, then antidepressants might help. Low doses of antidepressants help to control the vasomotor center in the brain that controls body temperature and perception of heat and cold.

If you feel a hot flash coming on, try drinking cold water, and take slow deep breaths. Anxiety about the hot flash can actually make it worse.

• • • • • • •

Q. What's the normal age for menopause? Will I start at the same age my mom did?

There's no normal, but 51 is the average age in the U.S., according to the National Institutes of Health. As for whether your mom's age is a predictor of the age you'll start menopause, it may be. A study from Boston University's School of Medicine found that there is some connection between the age at which your mother went through menopause and the age at which you will. It was especially true for mothers and daughters who had unusually early or late menopause. Don't know when your mother started "the change?" Ask her—it's not need-to-know information, but I'm all for any question that gets you talking about your family health history.

Q. I've never had a problem with body odor in my life but my husband says I do now. What's going on?

There are two types of sweat, and they both do the same thing: regulate your body temperature and cool you down when you're getting too hot. The first comes from the sweat glands that are all over your body. This sweat contains salt and water and has no odor.

The other type of sweat, which is produced from sweat glands under your arms, around your genitals, and on your scalp, is different in that it contains fat and protein, which bacteria love to eat. When bacteria digest this sweat, they produce an odor—the typical body odor we all know and love (or not so much love).

When we enter perimenopause and menopause, these glands kick into overdrive as a result of the fluctuating levels of estrogen and progesterone. Plus, hot flashes make us sweat. More perspiration means more for the bacteria to eat, and thus more smell.

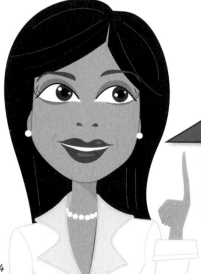

PSST, FROM DR. RAJ!
If your doctor recommends an invasive test or procedure (like removing an ovarian cyst instead of monitoring it for changes), and you're not sure it's right for you, ask what the alternatives are. It's good to know all your options and weigh them carefully before you decide what to do.

Don't worry. The sweat (and the smell along with it) will fade and most likely go away completely as your hormone levels adjust. Until then, ask your doctor for a prescription antiperspirant. It'll help prevent sweating so there's nothing for the bacteria to eat. Also, be sure to wear breathable fabrics (like cotton or supplex nylon in workout gear) as they help wick away moisture and keep bacteria from growing.

• • • • • • •

Q. I've been so dry down there lately that lube doesn't even do the trick. What else can I try?

Topical estrogen can be very helpful for this problem, which is most likely due to decreased estrogen levels. It works to heal vaginal tissue, restore moisture, and relieve discomfort. You can get it in a cream (Estrace, Premarin) or tablet (Vagifem) that is inserted into your vagina every night at bedtime. Estrogen-releasing rings (Estring) are also an option. They are inserted into your vagina (by you or your doctor) and are replaced every three months. Ask your gyno about this and other possible solutions at your next appointment.

Worried about using estrogen? There are estrogen-free moisturizers made just for the vagina (Replens or K-Y Liquibeads). They're over-the-counter but you should get your gyno's advice on which she thinks is best. A word of warning: Do not take the word "moisturizer" as a sign you can use any moisturizer. Regular lotions with moisturizers can be very irritating to your vagina. And just for good measure: Skip scented soaps, bubble baths, and douches. They will make the problem and discomfort worse.

Not near menopause? Breastfeeding, autoimmune disorders, and even your allergy medicine can cause this problem. Brainstorm with your doctor to find a solution.

In La La Land

chapter

7

Health styles of the rich and famous

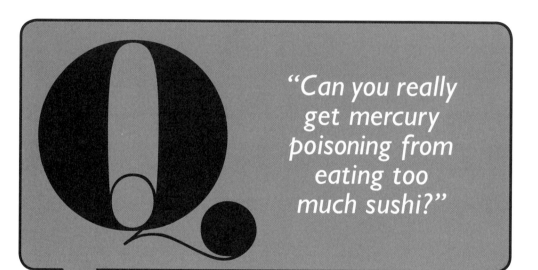

"Can you really get mercury poisoning from eating too much sushi?"

Believe it or not, you can. Mercury—a toxic heavy metal that can cause neurological problems—exists in high levels in such sushi staples as tuna (bluefin is one of the worst), mackerel, yellowtail, swordfish, and sea bass. (Other fish can contain a lot of mercury if they swim in polluted waters.) So if you're eating sushi (particularly these bad-news varieties of it) more than six times a week, you could be getting too much mercury, as actor Jeremy Piven claimed he was.

I had a patient who came to me after surviving a heart attack. His doctor had told him to eat a high-fish diet, so he dutifully grilled tuna every day for a year. Then, he started noticing weird neurological symptoms. We tested his mercury level and it was through the roof.

So how can you detox your sushi platter? First, don't eat fish every day. If you're going to have seafood that often, at least cut back on the most mercury-filled varieties. Skip these types of fish entirely while you're pregnant or nursing, because mercury exposure can very seriously harm the development of a fetus or young child. And don't serve it to your little ones, who can be affected by much lower levels of the metal than adults would. (In fact, very young kids shouldn't eat raw fish period because of the risk of food poisoning, which can be devastating.) And if you start to experience symptoms such as tremors, vision problems, and irritability, or if you just want to know you're in the clear, ask your doctor for a blood-mercury check. If it's high, he may advise you to cut back.

THE MOST TOXIC TAKEOUT

Ordering in sushi? Pass up these mercury-rich fish.

1. Bluefin tuna

2. Other varieties of tuna

3. Swordfish

4. Mackerel

5. Sea bass

• • • • • •

Q. When celebs are hospitalized for exhaustion, what do they have exactly?

You got me! "Exhaustion" is not a medical diagnosis, and it's certainly not one for which you will be admitted to any legit hospital.

It is true that if you *really* overtax your body—by abusing alcohol or drugs, not sleeping for days on end, starving yourself, or undergoing extreme physical stress (as you might experience doing your own stunts or filming in a remote location), you can wear yourself out and suffer physical symptoms as a result. Basically, your body starts to act up. Your immune system may get weak, making you more prone to infections—particularly viruses like the one that causes mononucleosis. You may become malnourished or dehydrated and need IV fluids or nutritional supplements. And you're more likely to suffer depression and anxiety, or their precursors—irritability and tearfulness.

So if a star gets the "exhaustion" label, it could be any or all of the above. Or she may just be wiped out. She checks into a clinic for a little R&R, while we may be more inclined to eat ice cream in our pajamas and watch Oprah!

3 Most Dangerous Health Tips from Celebs

Do yourself a big favor and tune out these public disservice announcements.

 DON'T VACCINATE YOUR KIDS. While it's laudable that celebrities want to raise awareness about autism (we still don't know what causes it, by the way), encouraging worried parents not to vaccinate puts tons of kids at risk of contracting serious preventable diseases like measles. Study after study has found there's no link between vaccinations and autism.

 SKIP TRADITIONAL CANCER TREATMENTS. Several celebs have revealed how "natural supplements" and "immune treatments" have helped them get over cancer. It sounds good, but there's not a shred of evidence that herbal treatments stop cancer. If you're living with cancer, you need traditional treatments that have been shown to work; if you want to add alternative remedies, do so under the supervision of your oncologist.

REVERSE MENOPAUSE SYMPTOMS WITH BIOIDENTICAL HORMONE REPLACEMENT THERAPY (BHRT). Some celebs have touted these as natural alternatives to traditional hormone replacement therapy (HRT). Only problem: Many bioidenticals are not Food and Drug Administration (FDA) approved, so there's no guarantee of what you're getting, or that they're safe or effective, let alone more so than conventional HRT.

Q. Is it true stars schedule their C-sections early so they don't get fat?

It is true, but I don't know how often it happens. And no matter the number who do or how fabulous the stars are, it's always a bad idea.

First of all, they're not saving themselves many pounds. Most of the weight you put on occurs earlier in the pregnancy. Toward your due date, you should only be gaining one or two pounds per week. In addition, this weight gain is very important—it helps ensure the healthy growth of the baby.

Second, recent studies show that delivering babies even as little as three weeks early can affect their health and learning abilities for the rest of their lives. Who would want to risk her baby's future to escape a few pounds of pregnancy weight? Plus, scheduling a C-section for convenience's sake is too risky for you and baby for lots of other reasons.

My bottom line: Anyone who has had a baby knows that the last few weeks are the worst in terms of physical discomfort (back pain, pelvic pressure, peeing all the time, heartburn), but it makes sense for your baby's health and yours to hang on to the end.

● ● ● ● ● ● ●

Q. So many stars pack on weight for acting roles, but is it dangerous to gain a quick 50 pounds and then lose it a second later?

You bet it is. Rapid weight gain can put stress on your heart and joints. Rapid weight *loss* can damage your liver and cause gallstones, hair loss (due to low protein), and loss of muscle mass; in starvation mode, your body hangs on to fat and breaks down muscle. It can also lead to loose, hanging skin, which— while not dangerous—is unattractive and hard to get rid of without surgery.

Of course, celebs are under a lot of pressure to shed their movie-part pounds in time for the next awards show, but no one should be speed dieting. One to two pounds per week is the fastest *anyone* should be losing weight. Even celebrities.

7: In La La Land

Q. Jennifer Love Hewitt said recently that she bedazzled her vajayjay after a break-up to feel better. Is it okay if I do it too?

I wouldn't recommend it. Using glue or any other sticky substance on your "vajayjay" is not a bright idea—though it may be a shiny one. Considering how sensitive the skin around your vagina is, gluing crystals only ups your chances of irritation and inflammation. Plus, as fun as it may seem to apply all those crystals, remember this: What goes on must come off. Can you imagine ripping them off one by one? Oh, the pain!

• • • • • • •

Q. How do celebrities have babies and then fit in their skinny jeans like four weeks later?

Well, we have to be honest here—most of these celebs you're thinking of (Gisele, Angelina, Halle Berry, and Heidi Klum come to mind) were pretty skinny and in great shape before their pregnancies. And most continued to work out regularly during those nine months. So if they are genetically blessed and have a healthy routine in place, chances are they're going to have an easier time than most dropping baby weight.

And keep in mind that these famous moms can afford daily sessions with personal trainers, live-in chefs whipping up healthy spa cuisine for every meal, home gyms that could rival any sports club, and 'round the clock childcare help so they can sleep and exercise when they want. With all that, you can see why they have a bit of an advantage over us mere mortals.

Remember, many of these women feel that their multi-million-dollar careers depend on them always looking their best, and if that means losing the weight ASAP, they do it. That's fine as long as women don't try to prevent

20

Percent that colonoscopies rose in the year after Katie Couric—who lost her husband to colon cancer—had an on-air screening in 2001. Good job, Katie!

Source: Archives of Internal Medicine

pregnancy weight gain by severely restricting calories and working out obsessively while expecting, since that can be harmful for the baby.

In the real world, six months is a more realistic goal for getting your body (almost) back. If it takes a little longer than that, that's perfectly fine. You're probably not stripping off your clothes for a love scene with George Clooney anytime soon, so there's no need to rush it. Enjoy your baby, and ease back into a healthy routine. The skinny jeans will come.

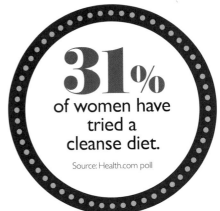

31% of women have tried a cleanse diet.

Source: Health.com poll

• • • • • •

Q. I recently read a celeb's blog about the importance of colon cleanses. How do I know if *my* colon needs cleansing?

Trust me, it doesn't. As someone who looks inside people's colons every day—yep, that's my job!—I can tell you that for most people, the colon does a perfectly good job of eliminating waste. It does not need any outside help to "cleanse" itself. In fact, colon cleanses might not be as "cleansing" as you'd hope. They can cause unpleasant side effects like abdominal pain or diarrhea. And if you have a chronic medical condition or are on medication, you shouldn't go there—the cleanse can make your condition worse.

If you feel like you're backed up in there, you can get things moving without having to try this extreme method. First tip: Eat plenty of fresh fruits and vegetables and drink a lot of water. Fiber supplements are another option. They add bulk to the stool, which helps move things out of your colon.

Still not getting the relief you want? Talk to your doctor. There might be another cause—like a thyroid condition or even a polyp—to explain your constipation. Just whatever you do, dump the cleanse. I promise you, it won't live up to the celeb hype.

7: In La La Land

Q. **Are celebs more fertile than the rest of us? How come so many are able to have babies in their mid and late 40s?**

You've stumbled onto one of Hollywood's "Dirty Little Secrets": donor eggs and in vitro fertilization (IVF). While being famous can get you far in life, it doesn't extend the warranty on your ovaries. It just gives that A-lister greater access to cutting-edge fertility treatments and doctors that the rest of us may not know about or be able to afford.

Starting in our late 20s and early 30s, the chances of conceiving naturally begin to go down (we have fewer and fewer eggs and their quality starts to decline). Then after age 35, the number of viable eggs falls off even more. So it's very difficult for any woman, celebrity or not, to conceive on her own after about age 40—at least with her own eggs.

And that's where IVF comes in. With IVF, an egg (often a donor egg if the mom is 40-plus) is fertilized outside the body and then transferred to the would-be mom's uterus. IVF can be very expensive and time-consuming, and it often requires multiple treatments.

In a perfect world, older Hollywood moms would talk openly about the time, money, and—oh yeah—younger woman's eggs it took to get pregnant. But big stars naturally want to keep these private reproductive choices under wraps. It's just too bad the rest of us end up getting the false idea that 40 is the new 20 when it comes to your reproductive system.

· · · · · · ·

Q. **The Duggars (from *19 Kids and Counting* on TLC) have 19 kids. Mom Michelle has given birth 17 times. How is her uterus not dragging on the ground?**

Back in the "good old days," women didn't have birth control, and they were giving birth and having more babies than we are now. Though few of us test

Nip/Tuck Scorecard

In Hollywood, it seems like every cosmetic tweak is popular. But what procedures are hot and not across the rest of the country? See below (numbers refer to the number of people having these procedures now vs. in 2007).

UP

HYALURONIC ACID (E.G. RESTYLANE) – 1,313,038 (2007 – 1 MILLION)

LASER HAIR REMOVAL – 1,280,031 (2007 – 729,000)

LIPOSUCTION – 283,735 (2007 – 269,000)

BOTOX – 2,557,068 (2007 – 4.3 MILLION)

BREAST AUGMENTATION – 311,957 (2007 – 348,000)

EYELID SURGERY – 149,943 (2007 – 206,000)

RHINOPLASTY (NOSE SURGERY) – 138,258 (2007 – 211,000)

ABDOMINOPLASTY (TUMMY TUCK) – 127,923 (2007 – 143,000)

MICRODERMABRASION – 621,943 (2007 – 713,000)

CHEMICAL PEEL – 529,285 (2007 – 940,000)

DOWN

the limits of our fertility anymore, our bodies are still capable of amazing things, like having 19 kids. Michelle Duggar is a prime example of that.

Of course, each pregnancy does take a toll on a woman's body. With each child and each passing year, it gets harder and harder to get pregnant, successfully carry the baby to term, and safely deliver the child. So at some point every woman has to say: Enough!

• • • • • • •

Q. Women like Kate Gosselin and the Octomom (Nadya Suleman) are birthing litters. How is that safe?

Every pregnancy carries some potential danger, and the risks increase with each successive pregnancy, especially if mom is older or has had previous C-sections.

With multiples (twins on up to octuplets), the danger—for both mom and baby—increases dramatically with each additional child. Kate's and Nadya's babies were born very young. Premature babies face a lifetime of possible health complications including asthma, learning disabilities, and vision problems. Also, in both cases, the moms were stuck in bed for several months before the deliveries because of the risks of a too-soon delivery.

Both moms used fertility treatments (Kate used intrauterine insemination and ovulation-inducing medications, and Nadya used in vitro fertilization), so their chances of having multiple pregnancies were high. While their high-risk pregnancies had a happy ending, it was potentially dangerous for all involved and could have gone another way.

91% of cosmetic procedures are done on women.

Source: American Society for Aesthetic Plastic Surgery

Q. Jessica Simpson posted a video on YouTube of her using an ear candle. I thought those were dangerous.

You're right—they are! Holding a burning candle near your face or ear or hair is never a good idea. There have been many reports of burns, middle ear damage, or eardrum perforation from this procedure. Also, the claims that burning a candle near the ear will magically draw out wax are simply not true. It doesn't work, and it's not worth the risk.

. . . . . .

Q. Salma Hayek recently breastfed a starving African baby. (The mother had no milk.) Is that okay?

Breastfeeding another woman's baby might confuse the baby. He is used to his mother's nipples, smell, and taste. He might have a hard time taking to you, or worse, he might not want to go back to his mom. Of course, it was better for Salma to have fed the baby than to let her starve.

Instead of pumping and donating breastmilk to an organization that sends it to starving children in Africa (yes, they really exist), better to donate money to a reputable non-profit that makes sure the mothers have proper nutrition. One good one is African Mothers Health Initiative (http://www.africanmothers.org).

HOW **BAD** IS IT *REALLY?*

To take diet pills to lose weight

Some prescription diet pills are okay, but the over-the-counter ones are risky. They can cause severe side effects like rapid heart rate and increased blood pressure, both of which raise your risk of heart attack. Plus, they usually don't work anyway…at least not like they promise. Don't go the drug route unless you're under the care of a good doctor.

Q. I want to try that maple syrup/cayenne pepper cleanse. Any precautions I should take?

Just one—don't do it! Your body does an outstanding job of cleaning up after itself. Instead of a Beyoncé-esque body, you might end up with abdominal pain or diarrhea, and weakness and muscle fatigue (from not having proper nutrients). Fact is, this kind of kooky cleanse can be just plain dangerous if you have a chronic medical condition. Let the stars have this one.

6 Celeb Health Heroes

These famous women used their star power to shine a light on oh-so-important health issues.

1972 | Former child star Shirley Temple Black goes public with the news she had a mastectomy, lifting the stigma about breast cancer.

1972 | Edith Bunker goes through "the change" in front of a live audience on *All in the Family*. She even says the word "menopause"!

1978 | Betty Ford admits she's addicted to painkillers and alcohol, and checks into rehab. Her honesty, as well as her first-rate treatment facility, helps countless women recover.

2005 | Melissa Etheridge, bald from chemotherapy treatments, performs at the 2005 Grammy Awards, empowering breast cancer patients everywhere to not feel ashamed.

2005 | Brooke Shields speaks openly about her postpartum depression, helping new moms understand that the condition is not a sign of weakness—or something they need to put up with.

2009 | Sarah Jessica Parker gets honest about her and hubby Matthew Broderick's troubles conceiving a second child. The couple decide to go with a surrogate and have a healthy set of twins.

Q. I heard lots of Hollywood stars start Botox in their 20s to *prevent* wrinkles. Does that approach really work?

Benjamin Franklin is quoted as having said, "The only things certain in life are death and taxes." I'd like to make an addition to that: wrinkles. If you smile, frown, or make any expression with your face (even squinting at the sun), you will develop laugh lines, brow lines, lines across your forehead, lines around your eyes, etc. They're a fact of life, and although there are ways to minimize them, we will all get them eventually.

It is true, though, that if you begin using Botox and fillers in your 20s, creases and wrinkles will be slower to develop. That doesn't mean they won't; it just means they will take some more time to show. Also, since these fillers are only temporary, you're signing yourself up for a lifetime of repeat treatments, at several hundred dollars a pop.

You can easily protect yourself from the biggest wrinkle maker: sun damage. I can't stress enough how much the sun destroys your skin day in and day out. Wearing a moisturizer with an SPF 30 will help keep the years (and wrinkles) from piling up on your face—no Botox needed.

PSST, FROM DR. RAJ!
If you're seeing a specialist, bring any prior test results or records with you. That saves you time and the cost of having to go get repeat tests.

Decode The Fillers

Does she? Doesn't she? Only her doctor knows for sure! But if you want a primer on how some women plump and fill, here's the scoop.

GENERIC: Botulinum toxinA
BRAND: Botox
WHAT IT IS: Not technically a filler, Botox is made from a protein in the bacterium *Clostridium botulinum*. It's the same toxin that causes botulism, a life-threatening type of food poisoning.
THE RESULTS: Botox blocks the signals your body sends to muscles, telling them to contract, thereby paralyzing the muscles. When the facial muscles can't contract, the skin stays flat, looking younger and less wrinkled.
WHERE IT'S USED: Mild to moderate facial lines, wrinkles, and creases
WHAT IT COSTS: $125-$400 a treatment
HOW LONG IT LASTS: Paralyzed muscles will begin functioning again in three to six months, so you'll have to repeat if you want to keep your skin wrinkle-free.

GENERIC: Collagen
BRAND: Zyderm and Zyplast (bovine-based collagen); CosmoDerm, CosmoPlast, Cymetra, Autologen, and Fascian (human-based collagen)
WHAT IT IS: Collagen is a natural protein in connective tissue.
THE RESULTS: As we age, collagen in our skin breaks down, leading to wrinkles. Collagen injections fill in wrinkles and creases.
WHERE IT'S USED: All over the face—from brow to lips. Many doctors will overfill the injection spot with collagen since 40 percent of the collagen will be absorbed very quickly.
WHAT IT COSTS: $300-$400 per syringe
HOW LONG IT LASTS: Collagen is eventually absorbed by the skin, so you may have to repeat the injections in three to six months to maintain the look.

GENERIC: Hyaluronic acid-based fillers

BRAND: Restylane, Perlane, Dermalive, Juvederm, and Hylaform

WHAT IT IS: These are natural carbohydrates that exist in human tissues.

THE RESULTS: These fillers work the same way as collagen, but results may last longer than collagen.

WHERE IT'S USED: All over the face—frown lines, crow's feet, lips.

WHAT IT COSTS: About $600 a syringe

HOW LONG IT LASTS: About six months

GENERIC: Synthetic poly-L-lactic acid (PLA)

BRAND: Sculptra

WHAT IT IS: It's a synthetic filler made from natural products.

THE RESULTS: Sculptra is designed for restoring volume and facial contours—either from scarring or severe wrinkles. Unlike Botox or collagen, PLA is diluted into sterile water, implanted in the skin, and then molded for aesthetics.

WHERE IT'S USED: Deep folds around the nose and mouth (smile lines), the lines framing your mouth (marionette lines), hollowed cheeks, and chin wrinkles.

WHAT IT COSTS: $450-550 per syringe

HOW LONG IT LASTS: You'll have four to six sessions to complete all your injections, but results last around two years. After that, you may need maintenance sessions.

GENERIC: Hydroxylapatite microspheres

BRAND: Radiesse

WHAT IT IS: It is particles suspended in a water-based solution.

THE RESULTS: Radiesse promotes your own body's collagen growth, filling in scars and plumping up wrinkles.

WHERE IT'S USED: Around the mouth and nose and in scars

WHAT IT COSTS: About $1000 a syringe

HOW LONG IT LASTS: About a year

All About Eating

chapter **8**

The skinny on food and dieting

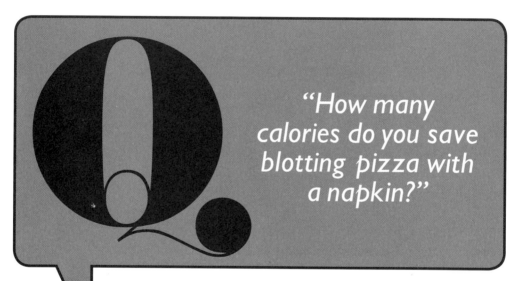

"How many calories do you save blotting pizza with a napkin?"

You are probably cutting 20 to 50 calories a piece—not a whole lot, but I guess if you have a couple of slices, it adds up. So if it makes you feel better, go for it.

Other ways to skinny up your pie: Ask the pizza guy to cut it into 10 or even 12 slices (each piece will have fewer calories and less fat), and start with a salad so you aren't famished by the time you open up that box. Also, order whole wheat or thin crust, avoid fatty toppings like sausage or pepperoni, and go for veggies like peppers or mushrooms instead. And, of course, if you skip the cheese, you'll cut out a whole lot of calories and saturated fat. But call me old-fashioned: It's just not pizza without any cheese.

Q. How long is it safe to stay on a juice fast?

Don't do it longer than one day. Our bodies need a varied diet—too much of any one food to the exclusion of everything else deprives us of the essential nutrients we need to function well. Drink only juice and you'll miss out on protein, healthy fats, and a slew of vitamins and minerals. Plus, healthy adults who swear off foods can suffer fatigue, headaches, constipation, and even heart rhythm irregularities. And certain people should never, ever fast (children, pregnant women, people with diabetes, kidney or liver disease, and anyone taking prescription drugs).

The proponents of juice fasting and other detox diets claim your body needs a "break" from digesting solid food in order to detoxify and help reset some sort of balance. As a GI doctor, I can tell you this is absolutely not true. Our kidneys and liver are responsible for removing toxins, and they do not react well to fasting. So that means your fast could actually prevent your body's natural detox system from doing its job. As for your digestive system needing a rest? False.

But let's be honest: The real reason most people try these extreme fasts is to lose weight fast. While you may knock off a couple of quick pounds on a juice bender, you're just losing water weight so those pounds will come right back. And let me tell you, a few days with less bloat is not worth risking potentially dangerous side effects.

* * * * * *

Q. Can high protein diets really mess up your kidneys?

High protein plans like Atkins may increase the risk of kidney stones, so anyone prone to stones or who has doctor-diagnosed kidney or liver disease should check with her doctor before trying a protein-rich diet.

Another problem with high-protein plans: They aren't very balanced, so you miss out on key foods your body needs like fruits, vegetables, and grains. Also, dieters on these regimens tend to eat way more red meats, salty foods like deli meats, and cheese—and thus get more saturated fat and cholesterol—than they normally would, putting them at risk for high blood pressure and heart disease. That's why many nutritionists now believe that the healthiest diet plans are ones that incorporate all kinds of whole foods, including—gasp!—healthy carbs like rice, beans, and pasta.

• • • • • •

Q. Food always smells fine to my husband, but funny to me. Why?

Chalk it up to the mighty female nose: We have a more sensitive sense of smell than guys do. Our internal odor-detector is strongest mid-cycle when estrogen is high (although birth control pills can dampen your sense of smell). And we're practically bloodhound-like when we're under the spell of pregnancy hormones. Think about it: How many of us first realize we're pregnant when we start being repulsed by ordinary odors (morning coffee, our husband's sneakers) that never bothered us before. This pregnancy superpower may have an evolutionary explanation, since being able to sniff out bad odors helps prevent you from eating something that could harm your fetus.

Is your guy older than you? The older you get, the weaker your sense of smell. Certain prescription medications, medical conditions like diabetes, and smoking can decrease his sense of smell, too. And keep in mind that in general people sense the same smells differently (why some of us love classic scents like heavy floral scents and others find them stinky). Your senses are there to guide you, so if food smells bad to you, it might not be spoiled, but heed your own schnoz and pass it up.

67%

That's how much your risk of becoming obese goes up if your sister becomes obese.

Source: New England Journal of Medicine

BY THE NUMBERS

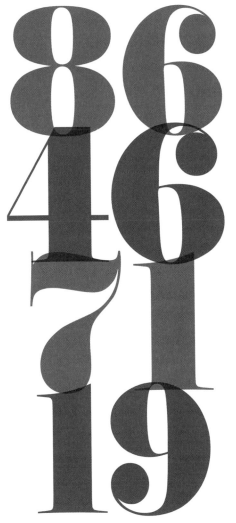

86% of women say they wait until they're alone to eat their favorite indulgent foods.

· ·

46% of women have been caught digging into a secret stash of food.

· ·

71% of women have buried a food wrapper deep in the trash to hide the evidence.

· ·

19% of women have snuck something off a friend or spouse's plate when he or she went to the rest room.

· ·

Source: Health.com poll

Q. **I love cupcakes, but the frosting gives me an instant headache. Why? Is this like an ice cream headache?**

Nope, it's a cupcake headache. What the heck is that? Probably a type of sugar headache—eating high-sugar foods leads to a rapid rise in blood sugar, which triggers a spike in insulin (a hormone that regulates blood sugar), which then causes a sudden drop in blood sugar. That can leave your head throbbing.

You get an ice cream headache, on the other hand, when the coldness of the yummy stuff causes the blood vessels in the roof of your mouth to contract and dilate.

Don't worry, you don't have to kick the confections. To combat the frosting headache, try eating your cupcake or cake a little at a time. Difficult, I know, since a cupcake practically begs to be popped into your mouth in one delicious bite. Adding nuts on top of your 'cake also may help, by regulating your blood sugar level. To avoid the Ben & Jerry's headache, sip some warm water or touch your tongue to the roof of your mouth to warm it (and prevent the contraction and dilation) between spoonfuls.

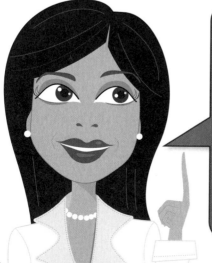

PSST, FROM DR. RAJ!
Make friends with your doctor's office staff. They often have all the control about who gets squeezed in last minute. And they definitely have favorite patients—namely, the ones who are respectful and don't take out their insurance-company frustrations on them. So do yourself a favor and get in good with them.

Q. **If a big pasta meal makes you tired, why do runners eat that before a marathon?**

It sounds counterintuitive, I know. Carbo loading before a major athletic activity (like running a marathon) is done so that the runner's body can maximize energy stores, helping ensure endurance and minimize fatigue.

Here's why carbo loading works: When we exercise, we slowly use up glycogen stores in our muscles and liver for energy. Once depleted, our muscles start to fatigue, but having extra carbs increases our glycogen stores and we can endure longer periods of high-intensity exercise.

Keep in mind that athletes who carbo load have that big plate o' carbs the night before, so their body has time to process and store them; they'd never sit down to a heaping stack of pancakes the morning of the race or they'd be pooped.

· · · · · · ·

Q. **I've been known to throw out forbidden foods and then fish them out of the trash. I know it's gross—but is it dangerous?**

It is indeed. That hunk of pie you just retrieved may have touched bacteria-laced raw or spoiled food (egg shells, old meat), which can make you very sick.

Also, it's a garbage can, so there could be metal or other non-edible objects hidden in the recently tossed treat. These hazards can enter your digestive system and cause internal damage. Every year people go to the hospital because they've inadvertently swallowed something like glass, razor blades, or bottle caps. Don't let that be you.

WHO KNEW?

Not getting enough zzz's may make the numbers on your scale creep up. Sleep deprivation leads to higher levels of the hunger hormone ghrelin and lower levels of a hormone that makes you feel full (leptin). This might explain why college students and new parents pack on the pounds.

3 Things That **Burn Fewer** Calories Than You'd Think

 PUSH-UPS: 272 cals for 30 minutes (and who can do push-ups for half-an-hour straight?)

 VIGOROUS SEX: 55 cals for 30 minutes

 GOLF: (walking and carrying your own clubs) 153 cals for 30 minutes

...and 3 That **Burn More**

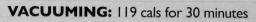 **PLAYING GAMES LIKE HOPSCOTCH WITH YOUR KIDS:** 170 cals for 30 minutes

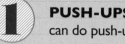 **INLINE SKATING:** 425 cals for 30 minutes

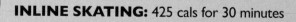 **VACUUMING:** 119 cals for 30 minutes

Q. Whenever I diet I get horrific bad breath. Why?

I'm guessing you're on a low- or no-carb diet. These plans cause your body to break down fat and release chemicals called ketones, leading to not-so-pretty breath. Try drinking more water to dilute the odor or chewing on mint leaves to cover it up. Adding back some carbs is the best way to permanently fix the problem.

If you aren't on a high-protein plan and notice a stench, you may simply be dehydrated and not producing enough saliva (saliva helps keep our breath fresh). Drinking more water should help, but if it doesn't, check in with your doctor. There's a chance you could have another problem like a respiratory infection, chronic sinusitis, or diabetes.

• • • • • •

Q. I sometimes use diuretics to drop a couple of pounds fast. Bad idea?

If you have to ask… Yes, very bad idea. Diuretics cause you to lose water and electrolytes (like potassium and sodium), leading to dehydration. This prompts your body to retain water—meaning you'll just pack back on whatever water weight you lost.

More bad news: Taking diuretics can bring on a dangerous drop in blood pressure. If you overuse them you can suffer kidney damage, and the loss of electrolytes can lead to abnormal heart rhythms.

You've surely heard it before, but having a long-term healthy eating plan and exercise regimen is a much better weight-loss strategy.

8: All About Eating

Q. I've been craving sweets lately—could that mean I have diabetes?

Nope. Craving sugar is not one of the symptoms of diabetes, or hyperglycemia (too much blood glucose). Symptoms to look for are frequent urination, excessive thirst, fatigue, weight loss, and blurry vision. If you skip meals often you may be experiencing hypoglycemia, or low blood sugar. When your blood sugar starts to dip, you naturally long for a sugary snack to get it back up. But the body processes sugar fast, so the energy surge quickly wears off and you're left craving another cookie.

Another common culprit? Low levels of serotonin, the brain chemical responsible for making us feel happy. If you have chronically low levels, your sugar yen could be your body's attempt to fix the problem—studies suggest that sugar increases the absorption of the amino acid tryptophan, which the body uses to make serotonin.

The good news: You can break the cravings cycle. First, stick to three or more healthy meals a day—no skipping! Blowing off a meal can cause your blood sugar to drop and your body to seek a solution—like a hit of chocolate or pint of coffee ice cream. Instead, choose good-news fare that keeps you satisfied.

And when you've just gotta have a little something sweet, just go right ahead. If you are at a healthy weight and not under a doctor's instructions to limit your sugar intake, there's really no reason you can't indulge—in moderation, of course!

TRUE OR FALSE?

Parasites can help you lose weight.

Well, having an intestinal parasite may make you thinner but it's a terrible idea for a diet! Parasites can give you diarrhea, severe abdominal pain, nutritional deficiencies, anemia, and lung and liver disease.

This Internet fad isn't a new idea, incidentally. Around the turn of the 20th century, advertisements for medicinal tape worms touted them as a weight-loss aid. If the thought of swallowing a live worm isn't disgusting enough for you (it's enough for me!), imagine seeing one come out of your rectum when you go to the bathroom. Or worse—when you are lying in bed. It takes a lot to gross me out, but this one definitely does.

Q. **How safe is it to eat those rotisserie chickens that sit under the heat lamps half the day?**

Although the heat lamps probably kill all harmful bacteria in the chickens, you never know if someone plucked that bird out from under the lamp, shopped for a while, and then changed her mind and put it back. In that case, it's possible some bacteria started growing.

Food shouldn't stay parked under those lamps for more than four hours, so check the time stamped on the container or ask the people behind the deli counter how long it's been sitting out. Also keep in mind that chains may cook up chickens that are just about to expire; sketchy grocery stores may even prepare the ones that are past their use-by date. In a pinch? Go ahead and grab that recently-cooked rotisserie. But I'd think twice about making these pre-made chickens a go-to meal.

* * * * * *

Q. **I like taking fish oil supplements for the omega-3s. The fishy burps they give me, not so much. Anything I can do to avoid that side effect?**

You're not the first to complain about popping an omega-3 pill and burping up sea smells all morning. Who wants to take a supplement—even one with amazing heart-health benefits—if it literally leaves a bad taste in your mouth? Here are a few easy strategies that should help:

Try a different brand. Cheap pills are made with cheap oil and may not come from reputable producers. Not only are they more likely to cause smelly burps but they also may contain unacceptable levels of toxins such as mercury. Ask your primary care doctor or pharmacist to recommend a reputable brand.

Scan the label. Your pill should be "pharmaceutical grade," meaning the oil is taken from healthy fish from

64%
of women have knowingly eaten expired foods.

Source: Health.com poll

clean waters, and is processed and purified in a high-quality facility.

Take it with breakfast. Sorry, but just coffee won't do if you're taking supplements. Pop that pill with a solid breakfast to ease stomach upset. Chew slowly, too, to avoid swallowing air, which causes burps.

Freeze your pills. They'll break down slower in your stomach, which means less gas and belching. Note: Some manufacturers advise against this, because the pills may lose some of their health benefits if frozen, so be sure to read the label and freeze accordingly.

If these moves don't help you, go the food route: You can get your omega-3 fix by eating more salmon, tuna, or walnuts, or from flaxseed oil pills (you can also sneak in flaxseed powder—which has a pleasant nutty flavor—by sprinkling it on yogurt). Common foods like orange juice and eggs are now fortified with omega-3s, too. Bonus: Your body may absorb the nutrients better when they come directly from food.

· · · · · ·

Q. Is it true I'll live longer if I eat every other day?

It is true that studies show this. It's also true that all the good studies were done on rats, mice, and worms.

That said, there is some evidence that severely restricting calories by eating every other day may prevent cancers and lengthen lifespan. However, the only study in humans was retrospective, meaning it looked back on a population that ate like this and then drew conclusions. In real-world practice, most of us would find this diet very tough to stick to, because it would make us tired and darn cranky on fasting days.

HOW **BAD** IS IT *REALLY?*

To eat a slice of bread that's in the same loaf as a piece that has mold on it

Best to toss the loaf. Bread is very porous, so mold can spread quickly, particularly in organic products that don't contain preservatives. Plus, mold has roots, so it could be thriving in microscopic amounts on slices that appear mold-free. The same goes for moldy meats, soft cheeses, jams, and fruits or vegetables. (Caveat: Fruit such as strawberries that has not directly come in contact with moldy pieces but are in the same container can simply be washed and eaten.) To avoid mold, keep food in a cool dry place or in the fridge. Always check expiration dates, too, and eat any leftovers within three days. Chances are you'll be fine if you do eat a tiny amount of moldy bread, though it could make you a little sick to your stomach.

Also, eating every other day would be dangerous for anyone with medical conditions and/or taking certain medicines. Instead of going to this extreme, just limit your calories enough to maintain a healthy weight—a proven and doable way to add years to your life.

• • • • • •

Q. My stomach is so sensitive that I'm afraid to eat out for fear that I'll end up in the bathroom all night. What can I do?

It's worth paying your doctor a visit sooner rather than later. But before you go, gather some information in a food diary: Write down everything you eat, when you eat it, and what seems to give your stomach grief. Even if you don't see a correlation, your doctor might.

One cause she'll surely consider is irritable bowel syndrome (IBS), a condition that, while still fairly mysterious to researchers, is very common, especially in women. It seems to be triggered by certain foods, as well as stress. IBS typically causes abdominal pain and diarrhea, bloating, or constipation. Even normal levels of stress can cause a flareup. If your doctor suspects this is your problem, she may recommend a laxative or fiber supplement depending on your particular symptoms. Or she may prescribe an antispasmodic medication or ask you to try probiotics (good bacteria supplements).

Your doc may also check for lactose intolerance (inability to break down dairy products), celiac disease (an allergy to gluten, a protein found in wheat), or other digestive diseases like an ulcer or colitis, a relatively rare condition involving inflammation of the colon. In some cases, cutting one food or food group out of your diet may do the trick. In others, either over-the-counter or prescription meds will be offered. If your doctor suspects an ulcer, she might schedule an endoscopy, which is a visual check of the upper digestive organs via a flexible, lighted tube inserted through your mouth.

The bottom line? You don't have to live with ongoing tummy troubles. Chances are you can find relief—and enjoy eating at restaurants without paying for it later.

Eat Red, Live to 100!

Well, not necessarily. But these crimson bites are
powerful anti-agers, according to research.

 RED CABBAGE has deep-red (almost purple)
pigments containing 36 plant chemicals that
researchers say may help guard against cancer,
boost brain function, and promote heart health.

 BEET JUICE contains a chemical that may help
reduce your blood pressure, according to British
scientists. Try mixing it into a smoothie.

 TOMATOES have lycopene and beta-carotene,
antioxidants that can keep your heart young by
lowering your bad cholesterol and increasing
your good cholesterol.

Knocked Up

chapter

9

With child—and
without a clue about
what's happening
to your body!

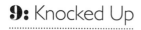

9: Knocked Up

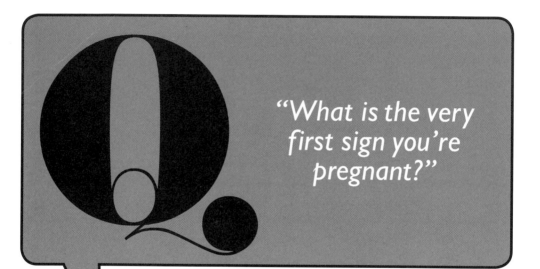

"What is the very first sign you're pregnant?"

Ask ten women their earliest sign and you'll hear ten different things. Some women experience swollen or tender breasts one to two weeks after conception. Others notice a darkening of the areola (the skin around the nipples). You may have nausea, headaches, or fatigue due to hormonal changes. Feeling faint and needing to pee more often can also signal early pregnancy.

You may also have food aversions or cravings or increased sensitivity to smells. A friend of mine knew something was up when a co-worker passed by her and she smelled the very strong scent of oranges. He had eaten oranges—several hours earlier! One pregnancy test later, her suspicions were confirmed.

And you should know: Slight vaginal bleeding could also be a sign; this spotting sometimes happens when the embryo implants into the uterus.

Q. Is it true certain positions give you a boy or a girl?

I wish I could say there was some magic position or special day in your cycle that yields a boy or girl, but the fact is it's the luck of the draw. Semen contains millions of sperm—half with an X chromosome and half with a Y chromosome. Whether you'll have a bouncing boy or a giddy girl in nine months is determined by which sperm (X or Y) reaches the egg and fertilizes it first.

Countless studies have looked for a relationship between sex positions and gender and come up empty. (Same goes for methods of timing sex around specific days in your cycle.) So no need to twist yourself into a pretzel...unless you want to, of course!

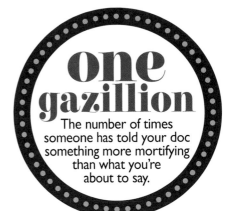

one gazillion
The number of times someone has told your doc something more mortifying than what you're about to say.

• • • • • •

Q. Before I knew I was pregnant, I worked on my laptop constantly. Could I have done damage?

Good news: You don't have anything to worry about. In the first few weeks of pregnancy, the fetus is so small that there is plenty of cushioning from the amniotic sac and uterus, so it's pretty well insulated from the pressure from your computer. (Also not a worry: radiation from computers, which used to be an issue but no longer is.)

But, starting now, I'd advise you to keep that laptop on a table. Some laptops can get very hot after awhile, and you don't want to overheat your abdomen or pelvic area. Also, having a heavy computer on your lap for long periods of time could interfere with the circulation in your legs.

Q. Why does an "innie" navel pop out when a woman is pregnant, but not if she just gains a lot of weight?

The growing fetus and uterus, and build-up of amniotic fluids cause your abdomen to expand rapidly when you're pregnant. So much pressure so fast stretches your skin and ultimately turns your "innie" navel into an "outie." During normal weight gain, however, the stretching is much more gradual, so there's no intense, outward push on the abdomen. If your transformed belly button alarms you, though, try not to panic. It should become an innie again in a few months post-delivery. On the off-chance that it doesn't (this happens infrequently), minor plastic surgery can restore your innie status.

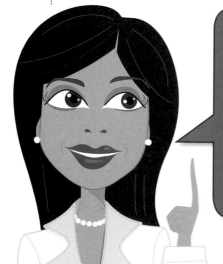

PSST, FROM DR. RAJ!
Go ahead and take a magazine into the exam room with you. Sometimes we get stuck with another patient, and you deserve to have something engrossing to read while you wait. Just put it down when the doc comes in—Brad and Angie will have to wait.

Q. I've heard that some women poop during childbirth. Please tell me it's not true!

Women love to tell gross and scary stories about labor and delivery, and this is one of the greats. Sure, it happens, but it's not all that common. In fact, many women have more bowel movements than usual the day before labor as their bodies prepare, so they're naturally "cleaned out" ahead of time.

It was once common for pregnant women to receive an enema before labor to empty their bowels; nowadays, most doctors skip the procedure. If you're really worried about this, you can request an enema at the hospital. But when push comes to shove in the delivery room, know that your doctor and nurses won't be the least bit fazed if a little poop escapes. They've seen it all before, and childbirth is naturally messy (though wonderful). Any poop will be whisked away quickly, no harm done.

• • • • • •

Q. Why do your feet grow after having a baby?

As you've discovered, your belly isn't the only thing expanding during your pregnancy. A pregnant body produces the hormone relaxin, which causes your pelvic ligaments and joints to loosen to make room for the baby's exit. That same hormone also relaxes the ligaments in your feet, allowing the bones to separate a bit. This, coupled with the fact that your increased weight puts more pressure on your foot arches, causing them to fall a bit, makes your feet grow. On average, you'll go up half a shoe size.

Plus, our feet tend to swell from retained fluids. Any change in size from fluid retention will disappear about a month post-delivery, but your new shoe size is here to stay. So don't celebrate getting preggo with a new pair of stilettos—you may need a bigger size in nine months.

TRUE OR FALSE?
If your mother had a hard time getting pregnant, you will too. **False.** Most causes of infertility are not hereditary—with the exception of endometriosis, which can be hereditary.

Q. I have to travel all the time for work. Could the airport screening devices harm my baby?

No. Although we don't want pregnant women being exposed to medical x-rays, the levels of radiation used in the airport screening machines, even the full-body ones, are quite low. Don't fret! They won't harm you or your baby in any way.

Many pregnant women worry about flying in general. But it's quite safe until around 34 weeks. After that, it is still safe to fly, but you risk delivering your baby in a strange city.

Also, since you are at increased danger of blood clots (from being pregnant and from flying), skip super-long flights. If you must fly across the globe, get up every half-hour or so and walk around to stretch your legs and keep blood flowing. If your pregnancy is anything like mine were, you'll probably have to use the bathroom that often anyway!

• • • • • •

Q. My husband is one of 5 boys. His father is one of 6 boys. Do we have even a *chance* of having a little girl?

Yes, despite the evidence you see in front of you (a family of boys), your chances of having a girl are 50/50. Well, okay, technically, 49/51. For some reason, the U.S. baby population skews to the boys—51 percent of babies are boys; 49 percent are girls.

When you examine any man's semen, regardless of his family history, there are equal numbers of X and Y chromosomes in the sperm. So don't paint the nursery walls blue yet—you could very well have an XX, aka a bouncing baby girl.

90%
of women say they've diagnosed themselves using the Internet.

Source: Health.com poll

Q. I've seen news reports of women having two babies by two different men at the same time. What in the world?!

This is extremely, *extremely* uncommon. These stories are in the news precisely because they are so rare!

Once you get pregnant, your body usually creates a mucus plug in the cervix to prevent any other sperm from getting through. Also, you stop ovulating. So if you have sex after you're pregnant, you won't have to worry about sperm fertilizing another egg.

But, in incredibly rare instances, a woman releases two eggs simultaneously and does not create a mucus plug. So she could get pregnant with two babies by the same man…or two different guys, depending on her social life!

• • • • • •

Q. Why does pregnancy make curly hair turn straight? Will mine go back to curly after I deliver?

Many women have the best hair of their lives when they are pregnant. The surge in hormones causes more of your hair to enter the "growth phase" and that means a thicker, more luxurious mane. Plus, you tend to eat healthier and take prenatal vitamins, too, so your hair gets glossier and stronger.

Those same hormones that give you Hollywood hair can also make curly hair straight or sometimes straight hair curly or wavy. Most of these changes go back to "normal" a few months after delivery (or after you stop breastfeeding).

HOW **BAD** IS IT *REALLY?*

To drink a glass of wine now and then while preggers

Bad. You may have heard that doctors in Europe don't ask their pregnant patients to stop drinking, just to cut back. Here's the problem with that approach: We don't know which women can safely have a glass of wine every now and then while pregnant without endangering their child, and which cannot. So if you drink at all while expecting, you're rolling the dice because you could be susceptible to passing on fetal alcohol syndrome or other developmental or neurological problems. And if you are, even one glass of wine may be too much. So to be safe, abstain completely. Putting off your next drink for nine months is a tiny price to pay to know your little one will be born free of a devastating brain disorder.

Q. During this pregnancy, my boobs have gone from a B to triple-D. How can that be normal?!

Do not fear your supersized ta-ta's. Most women will grow a cup-size or two, but increasing more is normal, too. Remember, your breasts are getting ready to provide milk for the baby, so your glandular tissue is increasing dramatically. Another reason for your expanding curves: You're likely retaining water. You may also notice darker and bigger nipples, darker areola (the skin around the nipple), more prominent bluish veins in your breasts, and increased breast tenderness.

If you don't like being a DDD, know this: You'll likely return to your normal size post-delivery (or after breastfeeding is complete).

But I should take this moment to stress the importance of good bras while you're pregnant. Bigger, more supportive bras can prevent back pain, and since you've already got lots of pains and strains everywhere else, invest in right-size, good-quality bras with wide supportive straps to hold up your new curves and prevent additional discomfort.

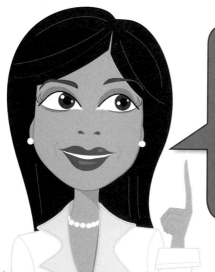

PSST, FROM DR. RAJ!
I never went anywhere without water while I was pregnant with my two sons. Your fluid balance shifts a ton when you are pregnant, which can lead to dizziness and lightheadedness, so always keep water on hand.

Q. I follow all the rules while pregnant, but I just can't quit eating Brie. How bad am I?

As a fellow Brie-lover, I am delighted to inform you that you don't need to give up your Brie (or other soft cheese like Camembert or goat cheese). But you do need to make sure that the cheese is pasteurized, so always, always check the label.

The danger in unpasteurized soft cheese is listeria, a type of bacteria that infects pregnant women more easily and severely than other people. Since it can cause stillbirths without any warning signs, don't ever chance soft cheese in a restaurant or deli where you have to take someone's word regarding pasteurization.

· · · · · ·

Q. Does eating Mexican food around your due date truly bring on labor?

Although I have friends who swear this is true, there is no medical evidence to support their stories. By the time that due date finally arrives, most women are so uncomfortable and desperate to go into labor they'll try anything—even an urban myth like eating spicy Mexican food. What makes these urban myths so compelling is we all know someone who tried it and then—surprise!—went into labor. But think about who tries these bring-on-the-baby tricks: Women who are at or past their due date! So they might have still gone into labor if they'd had Chinese food, or even broiled chicken, instead of chimichangas.

The truth is, there is no way to rush the process. Babies come out when they decide it's time. So eat all the Mexican food you want. You may not get a baby at the end of the night, but enjoying some chips and salsa should take your mind off your burning desire to get that kid out of you already!

What to Pack When You're Popping Out a Baby

Loading up your bag for the hospital?
Here are four things you don't want to forget:

 SNACKS: After the physical exhaustion and hours of starvation involved with labor, you deserve a major treat, and hospital food just doesn't cut it. So bring some of your favorite cookies, crackers, and juices.

 ROBE AND SOCKS: It could be the middle of summer, but hospital rooms are always cold. Keep cozy with socks and a robe.

 YOUR OWN PILLOWCASE: The feel (and smell) of your own pillowcase will be oh-so-comforting, and between visitors, you can get some shut-eye—the last you will have for a long time!

 GRANNY PANTIES: Whether you're having a C-section or a vaginal delivery, toss in your biggest pair of loose cotton undies. You'll need something that won't hit or irritate the scar (C-section) or your sore vagina (vaginal delivery), which is why your usual skimpy lacy pair won't fit the bill.

A. B. (After Baby)

Q. **My doctor told me I could resume sex after six weeks, but oh the pain! I'm as dry as the Sahara down there! Will it ever feel good again?**

Yes, yes, yes! Your dryness is a temporary and very common side effect of having a baby. The culprit: low estrogen. But don't worry, your hormones should be back to normal about six months after delivery. If you're breast-feeding, the dryness will usually last until you're finished because estrogen remains low until you wean the baby.

I hope you don't feel you must get busy at exactly six weeks just because it's medically safe to do so. Every woman is different, and you're the best judge of when you're ready. So if it hurts, wait a little before trying again. When the time is right, be sure to use lots of lube, so you don't end up with any abrasions or tears, which could be extra painful while that area is still recovering from childbirth. Also, to get good and lubricated, try to take time for foreplay (no easy task with a newborn in the house, I know). The most important tip? Give it time. Sex will feel great again. Promise!

· · · · · ·

Q. **I just stopped breastfeeding my baby, and now my once-full boobs look like collapsed baggies. Please tell me this is only temporary!**

Well, there's good news and bad news. First the good: This half-filled water balloon look is more or less temporary. After you stop breastfeeding, you undergo something called breast involution—the milk-making tissues that grew and expanded during pregnancy are now shrinking. The skin on your breasts takes a little longer to catch up—hence, the "baggie" look.

Within a few months, your breasts will develop more fatty tissue to fill them back up, and they will look more like your pre-pregnancy breasts (just don't expect them to be exactly the same).

Now for the bad news: The sagging, which occurs because the weight of your breasts during pregnancy and breastfeeding stretches the ligaments supporting them, will not reverse itself. Your girls will regain some of their elasticity—just not all of it.

In the meantime, go get fitted for a new bra. Wearing one that's the right size and gives the right support is essential for supporting the ligaments so they don't stretch as much. This should cut down on additional sagging.

● ● ● ● ● ●

Q. Is my vagina all stretched out now that I've given birth?

Repeat after me: A woman's body is a beautiful, amazing thing. This is never more true than during childbirth, when your vagina, by design, stretches and shrinks like an accordion. Better yet, giving birth increases blood flow to the area—temporarily for most, long term for some. And that's a very good thing for sensation.

On the other hand, many women find their pelvic-floor muscles are weaker post-delivery, which can cause urinary incontinence and even decreased sensation during sex. Not to worry: You can get those muscles back into shape with Kegels. To do these exercises, imagine you're sitting on a marble and must lift it off the chair using only your trusty vagina. Tense that area, hold for 10 seconds, and relax for 10. Aim for 10 to 15 Kegels three times a day. If you continue to experience pelvic-floor weakness, a physical therapist may be able to suggest additional moves. Surgery to lift the muscles in that area is an option, too, as a last resort.

1 in 3
babies in the U.S. are born by C-section. That's a 53% increase over the last decade.

Source: National Center for Health Statistics

Q. Is it true that there are weights you can insert in there to whip it back into shape?

Strange but true! You can pump up standard Kegels using vaginal weights. The weights were developed to help women with incontinence strengthen the pelvic muscles. You insert these tampon-sized "vaginal cones" into your vagina twice a day for 15 minutes. Start with the lightest weight, and after you're able to hold that in success-fully, advance to the next weight. Ask your doc to recommend a product that's right for you. That said, if you'd rather not pump iron down below, experiment with new positions: Changing the angle may just hike the amount of pleasurable friction for you and your man.

67% of babies are breastfed at least once in their lives.

Source: National Center for Health Statistics

• • • • • •

Q. After having a baby by C-section, I am totally flatulent. What's up with that?

All that gas is a side effect of weakened muscles and nerves in your pelvis and rectum, which makes it harder to control gas. Believe it or not, you were probably just as gassy before the baby, but it's much more noticeable now because you can't keep it in. Lucky you.

In one respect, you're better off than someone who delivered vaginally. One reason for difficulty holding in gas: anal sphincter injury as a result of tearing during delivery. You don't have to deal with that problem! But you did still stress your pelvic muscles during the pregnancy, so in that regard, we're all the same.

Controlling the gas should get easier as your muscles naturally gain strength again. Kegel exercises may be a big help. Oh, and cut way back on uber-gassy fare like beans, cabbage, onions, and sodas.

9: Knocked Up

Q. Why does breastfeeding make me feel turned on?

While your little one nurses, your body pumps out a cocktail of hormones that helps you two bond. These hormones, prolactin and oxytocin, affect your body and mind, making you feel relaxed, happy, and super-close to your baby. You may notice nipple tingling and sensations similar to what you feel during arousal and orgasm (oxytocin is also released during orgasm). Don't worry; that's perfectly normal. What you're experiencing is an overwhelming feeling of closeness with your baby, part of which is the satisfaction of knowing you're providing the best possible nutrition for your tiny one.

• • • • • •

Q. I have hideous stretch marks. Can you make them go away?

If I could, I'd be a rich woman. Almost 90 percent of us have stretch marks. Despite claims made on late-night infomercials, no cure-all lotion or cream will reliably erase those marks, which appear when skin stretched by the rapid growth of pregnancy (or major weight gain or loss) doesn't snap back. The marks start out red or purple, and fade to white over time. Your best bet for diminishing them is seeing a board-certified dermatologist for micro-dermabrasion or a chemical peel, procedures that slowly remove layers of the scarred skin tissue. Most derms suggest six treatments on any spot that needs work, which can cost $75 to $600 a session, depending on the treatment.

Hoping to prevent stretch marks? There's a limit to how much you can do, and some of it comes down to genetics. Plus, you can't help but stretch in pregnancy. Staying hydrated and exercising regularly improves circulation to your skin to maintain elasticity. As for all the belly rubs marketed to pregnant women for stretch mark prevention? Some women swear by them, but there's not yet scientific evidence to show they work. Lotions that contain cocoa or shea butter, olive oil, and vitamin E help your skin retain moisture, which may relieve the itching that accompanies dry skin and stretch marks.

Q. My husband wants to taste my breast milk—isn't that weird?

Well if it is, then most of the dads out there are weird. Almost every father I know has at least wondered what our milk tastes like.

Think about it—your husband has just gone from #1 guy in your life (and the one most familiar with your breasts besides you) to low-guy-on-the-totem-pole. Your baby is your all-encompassing priority right now, and your husband watches as your baby greedily guzzles from your breasts.

So it's normal for Dad to wonder what it's all about, and if giving him a tiny taste will satisfy his curiosity, then by all means, let him taste. But that's baby's only sustenance, so if Daddy wants more milk, tell him to go to Whole Foods (for the cow variety!).

• • • • • • •

Q. My friend wants us to breastfeed each other's baby? Is that even safe?

Breastfeeding is an incredibly special bonding experience between you and your baby. Why would you want to share that with anyone else besides your little one? Plus, swapping boobs might confuse him. He is used to you—your smell, your voice, your shape and size, and even the taste of your nipple. He may not want to suck from another breast; if he does try it, he may not want to go back to yours.

Also, many drugs, both legal and illegal, alcohol, and some infectious diseases (like HIV and TB) can be passed through breast milk to your baby. I personally would not trust anyone else to feed my baby. Especially a friend who would make a suggestion like this—she sounds nutty!

TRUE OR FALSE?

Can you get pregnant while breastfeeding?
True. While you are generally less fertile while you nurse, you are not infertile—especially if you are not exclusively breast-feeding (i.e. using some formula). So don"t let that lack of monthly periods fool you—you can still get pregnant and should use a birth control method (talk to your doc about which one) if you do not wish to become pregnant.

In Your Head

10

Moody, stressy, spacey: what's normal and what's not

10: In Your Head

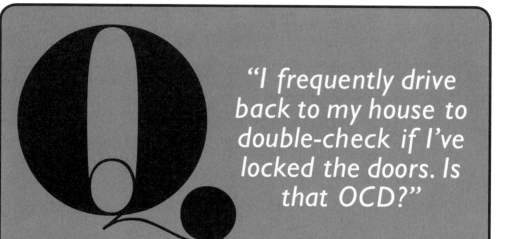

"*I frequently drive back to my house to double-check if I've locked the doors. Is that OCD?*"

Unlikely, but possible. People with obsessive-compulsive disorder (OCD) have both intrusive obsessions (fears of terrible things happening, like leaving on the stove and torching the house, for instance), as well as compulsive rituals—repetitive acts like checking and re-checking to make sure the stove was turned off—to calm those fears. Let's face it: A lot of us are a little obsessive and a bit compulsive. It's not OCD unless the behaviors really interfere with your ability to function, consume a ton of time, or cause you significant stress.

If your only OCDish behavior is rechecking your lock, and you're not obsessing about it that much of the time, you're probably okay. But since OCD does affect two to three percent of the population (pretty common as far as diseases go), if you are concerned about it you should speak to a psychiatrist: Both psychotherapy and medications may ease OCD symptoms.

Q. My heart sometimes feels like it's racing in my chest—am I having a panic attack?

Anxiety can definitely cause palpitations (feeling like your heart is pounding or jumping in your chest). If you are about to do something nerve-wracking like give a speech, you may feel your heart beating a little faster, which is a normal response to stress hormones.

True panic disorder (aka panic attacks) is a form of anxiety disorder that occurs for no discernible reason. So if you get these symptoms only when you have something stressful going on (a blind date, a public speaking engagement), it's not a panic attack but a case of nerves. However, if the chest symptoms come out of nowhere and you also feel intense fear or dread, feel faint, and are short of breath, trembling, or sweating, you could have panic disorder.

If you haven't been diagnosed with the disorder, get your symptoms checked out by a doctor. A racing in your chest could also mean there is something wrong with your heart—an abnormal rhythm, a heart valve problem, a heart muscle problem—all of which can be very dangerous if not diagnosed and treated. Your doctor will probably give you a test called a Holter monitor where you wear a machine for 24 hours that continually records your heart rhythm and rate; it's a continuous EKG. Assuming your ticker is fine, ask for a referral to a therapist because panic disorder is one of the most treatable anxiety disorders. Options include talk therapy, prescription medication, including antidepressants or sedatives, or a combination of meds and psychotherapy.

who knew?

The most prescribed drugs in the U.S. are antidepressants.

Source: Centers for Disease Control and Prevention

Q. Lately I've been blanking out on everything (friends' names, what I need at the grocery store). Could it be early Alzheimer's?

I wouldn't worry. There are many reasons why we become forgetful at times—stress, lack of sleep, certain medications (like sleep aids), depression, alcoholism, or even a vitamin deficiency (particularly B12). Even normal aging will produce some minor forgetfulness.

If you find yourself getting lost or forgetting how to get somewhere you go almost every day (like work or the grocery store) or if you notice you've forgotten how to do something like write a check or add numbers, then you have cause for concern. But blanking on someone's name? If that's Alzheimer's, everyone has it. Early-onset Alzheimer's (meaning the disease develops before age 65) is very rare—only five to ten percent of people with Alzheimer's disease are early cases. And symptoms before 50 are even more rare. So unless you're noticing extreme memory deterioration, or you have a family history of early-onset Alzheimer's, I wouldn't worry.

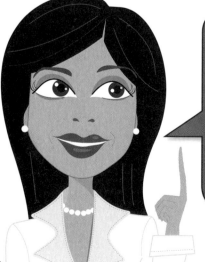

PSST, FROM DR. RAJ!
Not sleeping well? Got no appetite? Stressed out of your mind lately? Bring it up to your doctor. She can explore whether there's a medical reason for your symptoms, and if not, give you a referral to a mental health specialist who can help.

Q. I'm terrified to fly, but is it safe to take anti-anxiety meds? What if we crash and I'm too zonked out to escape?

In a panic about your anti-panic med, huh? Actually, you raise a good point. If you plan to take an anti-anxiety medicine before an important or stressful occasion, it's best to try it out well before the big day to see how your body reacts to it. Otherwise, you could end up like the bride who slept through her big day because she tried an anti-anxiety drug for the first time the morning of her wedding! Doing a trial run on the drug helps you and your doctor figure out what dose of the sedative is enough to keep you calm but still capable.

In general, it's better to try relaxation methods like deep breathing, yoga, or meditation before you reach for the drugs. But if you're truly a wreck about flying, an anti-anxiety pill may be right for you (avoid sleeping pills, though, which will leave you too out of it to spring into action if needed). Remember that the effects of meds like Xanax, Klonopin, or Valium can last for 24 hours so you shouldn't be the one driving that rental car out of the airport. And you can't drink while taking them (having cocktails on a plane is a bad idea anyway, because it makes you dehydrated).

HOW **BAD** IS IT *REALLY?*
To take a friend's Ambien

This is a big fat no-no. Taking someone else's prescription drug is *always* a bad idea. These drugs require a prescription for a reason: They have potentially serious side effects and may have a dangerous interaction with a medicine or vitamin you're already taking. An MD needs to consider all of these factors to determine if it's the right drug for you.

By the way, use caution with Ambien if you have liver or lung disease, depression, or drug dependence. Also, no driving within 12 hours after taking it if it's your first dose. Why? People sometimes black out with Ambien and actually drive somewhere without remembering it.

Q. How do I know if I'm really depressed or just extra cranky?

Depression is more than just feeling down or crabby. It's caused by a chemical imbalance in your brain that usually affects your mind *and* body. So while feeling sad or blue is one sign of depression, there are usually other physical clues like changes in appetite (usually loss of appetite), insomnia, frequent tearfulness, and extreme lethargy. You may also stop enjoying activities you used to love. As long as your cranky mood isn't causing problems at home or at work, or interfering with your ability to get through your daily activities, it's probably not depression.

We don't know exactly what causes depression, but many people with the disorder have lower levels of neurotransmitters, or brain chemicals that are directly linked to mood. Most doctors will prescribe selective serotonin reuptake inhibitors (SSRIs), like Prozac or Wellbutrin, or serotonin and norepinephrine reuptake inhibitors (SNRIs) like Effexor or Cymbalta, to increase neurotransmitters. Talking to a mental health professional may help, too.

Just remember, there's no reason to suffer. Depression is a real illness, and thankfully there are now good treatment options for it.

35%
of women have Googled to see if they're crazy

Source: Health.com poll

Q. Why do I feel magically better the day I get in to see the doctor?

Murphy's Law. Sometimes worrying about a symptom makes you experience it more and going to the doctor reassures you because you know it will be taken care of, or at least you will find out what is going on. Or it could be you're so scared of having tests done that you convince yourself that your symptoms are gone. Either way, don't break your appointment. Your doctor isn't just interested in how you are feeling that day, but rather the whole history of your problem.

How To Go There With Your Doctor

4 ways to make spilling your secrets easier

1) REMEMBER IT'S NOT A DATE. You don't have to make steady eye contact or worry that you're making a good impression. And if your doc is too handsome or cool for you to confess something embarrassing, he's probably not the right MD for you.

2) BE A REGULAR. If you're seeing your physician for yearly checkups and physicals, you're more likely to develop a comfortable tell-all relationship.

3) PREPARE TO STRIP. No matter what you're going to the doc for, assume you'll end up in that dreaded paper gown. If being half-undressed makes you feel weird, do whatever you need to do to get comfy. Wear clean underwear and shave your legs (it doesn't matter at all to us docs, but sometimes patients feel more relaxed when they're not self-conscious about their appearance).

4) SAY IT YOUR WAY. Your doctor doesn't care whether you tell her, "I have rectal bleeding" or "Yikes, I saw blood in my poo!" So don't worry about how you'll sound explaining your symptoms. And if you'd rather not say it aloud, feel free to hand her a list of questions/concerns. Or bring along a friend or a family member to help you feel more comfortable getting into the nitty-gritty details.

Q. **If alcohol is a depressant, why does a glass of wine take the edge off my bad days?**

Here's what's confusing you: The word "depressant" refers to what alcohol does to your central nervous system, not what it does to your mood. When alcohol first enters your bloodstream and gets to your brain, it causes you to lose some inhibitions and relax, and may slightly elevate your mood. But if you drink more than a couple of drinks, the depressant nature of alcohol really kicks in, meaning it slows down the activity of your brain. It may, in fact, make you sad or anxious. It can also make you confused, lethargic, and even comatose if you drink enough. One single glass of wine is the way to go: You get the health and mood perks without the depressant qualities.

Decode The 3 Vus

JAMAIS VU - "never seen"; forgetting how to do something you've done many times before; momentarily not recognizing a word, person, or place you've seen already. This can be part of epilepsy or another brain disorder.

DÉJÀ VU - "already seen"; this is that feeling you've experienced something before. Scientists say it's most likely not an act of "prophecy" but may happen when your brain takes in something new and records it as if were already a memory.

PRESQUE VU - "almost seen"; this is the "tip-of-the-tongue" syndrome, when you're searching for a word or answer but can't quite seem to get it out.

Q. I think antidepressants would help me, but I worry about the stigma if anyone finds out.

Unless you tell someone, the chances of anyone finding out are almost nil. Still, many people share your concern: More than 60 percent of employees think their status at work would be harmed if it was known that they had sought treatment for depression, a new survey from the American Psychiatric Association suggests.

But leaving depression and anxiety untreated is not a good idea. Untreated mild depression often gets worse and leads to an episode of major depression years later, according to Columbia University research.

If you're frequently feeling down, first talk with your doc. Increasing how much you exercise is an easy way to hike feel-good endorphins. If that isn't enough, combining therapy with antidepressants may help relieve depression better than meds alone, according to a major research review in the *Journal of Clinical Psychiatry*. If you do try the drugs, take pride in the fact that you're taking care of yourself—a sign of strength, *not* weakness.

70% of people have experienced déjà vu. It seems to be most common in early adulthood.

• • • • • • •

Q. I always feel like my mind's going in a million directions. Should I ask my doctor for Attention Deficit Disorder medicine?

Whoa, slow down! In this era of smartphones, BlackBerries, instant messages, and 24/7 news streaming, all of us at times feel distracted, pulled in a zillion different directions, and unable to concentrate. But with ADHD (attention deficit/hyperactivity disorder) this inability to focus, follow through, and complete tasks is pervasive enough to disrupt your life in many ways. Many people with ADHD have trouble in their careers, quitting out of boredom or getting fired over and over again. They also have trouble

6 Foods That Fight Off Bad Moods

 STEAMED EDAMAME: Folate-rich foods like edamame may even out moods, according to a few studies.

 YOGURT + GRANOLA: Protein increases the brain's dopamine levels, helping you feel more alert. And complex carbs provide long-lasting fuel for an energy burst.

 POPCORN: Rich in carbohydrates (and whole grains!), which stimulate the release of serotonin, popcorn also provides protein for a great afternoon pick-me-up.

 SUNFLOWER SEEDS: This yummy snack is a great source of magnesium, which regulates and improves your mood. Just one cup provides more than half of your daily magnesium requirement.

 BANANAS: This feel-great fruit gives you a sustained energy boost and is packed with vitamins and mood-boosting tryptophan to keep you happy longer.

 OATMEAL: Its healthy carbs help your body pump out serotonin, which makes you feel happier.

focusing on relationships. Other symptoms include impulsivity, restlessness, and being quick to anger. Since ADHD starts in childhood, your doctor can ask you a lot of questions about your symptoms and childhood to determine whether you have ADHD. She'll also consider other conditions that can cause trouble concentrating, including depression, lack of sleep, or even conditions like Lyme disease. If she thinks you do have ADHD, she may prescribe medication (such as stimulants like Concerta or Adderall) as well as counseling.

• • • • • • •

Q. I keep hearing how everyone these days is narcissistic. How do I know if I am?

The fact that you are asking probably means you don't have narcissistic personality disorder, because people who do have it generally don't have enough self-awareness to question their own behavior. While many people occasionally exhibit "narcissistic traits" like self-absorption or arrogance, true narcissistic personality disorder takes it to another level. People with this disorder have a very inflated image of themselves (exaggerating their talents), and expect everyone around them to admire them. They are very sensitive to criticism, believe others are jealous of them, and often have dramatic mood swings and outbursts. They also have a sense of entitlement. Behind the arrogant front, though, they usually have a self-esteem problem. Not surprisingly, celebrities in general and reality TV stars in particular rate super-high in narcissistic traits, according to a study by Dr. Drew Pinsky, MD, host of *Celebrity Rehab* and *The Mirror Effect: How Celebrity Narcissism is Seducing America.*

NOT TO WORRY!
Feeling grief after the death of a pet is normal
One-third of people who lose pets are in mourning for six months or longer, according to the Harvard Mental Health Letter.

Q. Is there really such a thing as a placebo effect? How does it work?

There is, and it's a fascinating bit of science meets psyche. When conducting research on a drug, scientists often split their study subjects into two groups. One group gets the real med; the other group gets a placebo—usually a sugar pill or other non-active medicine that looks just like the real drug so the participant and researcher won't know who's getting what.

What tends to happen is some of the people who get the sugar pill feel better. Since they didn't take any real medicine, they clearly weren't benefiting from an actual remedy. Instead, the power of suggestion kicked in: The fact that they thought they were getting medicine actually made their symptoms less noticeable. (Another explanation: Their problem just coincidentally went away, which is not an example of the placebo effect.) If you like and trust doctors, you're more likely to notice the placebo effect working for you. Bottom line: We sometimes feel better because we think we're getting medicine and should be feeling better (this also may be why some of us swear echinacea or vitamin C cures a cold, when research doesn't show it does).

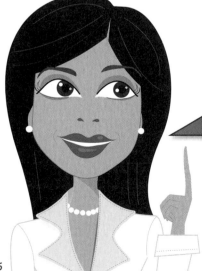

PSST, FROM DR. RAJ!
Got something rather private to discuss with your doc? If you're too embarrassed to spill while you're half-naked, ask to chat in her office before you strip down for the exam.

Psychologist vs. Psychiatrist

What the heck's the difference? Who is better?
Here's a quick primer:

PSYCHOLOGISTS have a doctorate (Ph.D. or Psy.D.), but in most states they can't prescribe drugs. They can treat patients who require mood medication, though; they work in tandem with psychiatrists who prescribe and monitor doses.

PSYCHIATRISTS are medical doctors, meaning they have completed medical school plus a residency. They can prescribe medication. If you have a serious and chronic mental illness like schizophrenia, you will likely be under the care of a psychiatrist rather than a psychologist or social worker. But many psychiatrists treat patients with much milder and temporary issues and do talk therapy as well as dole out drugs.

You can also receive therapy from a clinical social worker (CSW)—they have master's or doctorate degrees in social work. Check your insurance plan's mental health provision to see whether it covers care provided by a social worker before going this route.

Gym Confidential

chapter

11

You'll never sit
butt naked in the
steam room again!

11: Gym Confidential

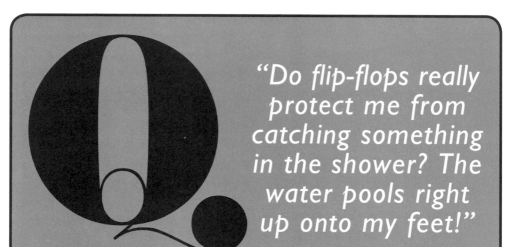

"Do flip-flops really protect me from catching something in the shower? The water pools right up onto my feet!"

Public shower stalls are hands-down the germiest place in the gym. The warm, moist environment makes them a dream breeding ground for bacteria and fungi. Flip-flops help a little bit, but you're right: If there are stagnant pools of water and you step in them, you might as well be stepping in barefoot! The thing you're most likely to catch is athlete's foot—a treatable but annoying fungal infection—but there are plenty of other nasty bugs out there.

Your gym should always be cleaning the showers (and the walls, which are equally gross) in between users. If you don't notice your health club doing this essential step, wait until you get home to shower off. But what if you're heading back to work or out and really need to wash up there? Avoid shower stalls with visible pools of standing water, don't touch the walls, and make it a quickie.

Q. **What's the worst thing you can catch from the machines at the gym?**

Probably the *worst* thing is the staph bacteria MRSA (short for methicillin-resistant *Staphylococcus aureus*), the "superbug" that can cause a very aggressive and difficult-to-treat skin infection, which can invade the blood. This bug, which is resistant to most kinds of antibiotics, is spread through close contact—athletes on a sports team sometimes spread it to each other. What's scary is it can survive on gym machines between users.

Wipe the equipment off with an antibacterial wipe before using it. And if you have any open sores or wounds or skin irritation, stay away from the machines because your broken skin will make you more vulnerable to contracting something.

54% of women have gone without flip-flops in the gym shower.

Source: Health.com poll

• • • • • •

Q. **Does wiping sweat off with just a towel do anything to protect from germs?**

Not a ton. It is true that moisture is the best place for germs to hang out, so wiping off any liquid on the machine will get rid of some germs, but bacteria and viruses can live on dry surfaces as well. The bug you're most likely to catch on that treadmill? The common cold, which can spread if you use a contaminated machine and then touch your nose, eyes, or mouth. (And how many times have you seen someone wipe their face before wiping off the equipment they're done with? Come on!)

Your best bet is to wipe it down with an antibacterial wipe. And always wash your hands after working out. That way, if you did pick something up on your fingers, you are less likely to contaminate yourself.

Q. Why do some people just smell worse when they're working out?

Gym BO is annoying—whether the stench is from you or the woman doing downward dog to your right. Sweat itself is odorless—it's what mixes with it (namely, bacteria) that causes the stink. Poor personal hygiene plays a big role—if someone hasn't showered in a day or two and has a lot of bacteria on her skin, she's gonna smell more. Hormonal changes, diet, and meds can also affect someone's bouquet. There are medical conditions that cause bad body odor, including diabetes, kidney disease, and fungal infections. If it's your problem, try the usual moves (frequent showering, applying antiperspirant before exercising) and if they don't work, talk to your doc. If you're offended by someone else's essence, keep in mind that she may not be able to help her odor. If the smell really bothers you, just scoot a few machines down.

• • • • • • •

Q. What's least germy: the sauna, steam room, or whirlpool?

Picture that scene in old horror movies where a mad scientist holds up a bubbling beaker full of some strange toxic brew. Just blow up the size of that beaker, and you have a whirlpool—a warm, bubbling cauldron of germs. It's the worst of the three, by far.

Interestingly, most of the bacteria hang out in the pipes, not the water. But when we turn on the jets, the germs are sprayed into the water. (If you own a hot tub, get the pipes professionally cleaned, and use a bleach disinfectant once a week for the tub. Remember—the hotter the water, the less effective a chlorine disinfectant is.)

Number 2 on the ick list: steam rooms. Warmth and extreme moisture is ideal for breeding germs. A sauna is number 3 on the list because the heat is dry. But any lingering sweat in the room is a moist habitat for germs.

who knew?

Intense aerobic exercise may suppress your appetite by reducing levels of hunger hormones in your stomach.

Top 5 Metabolism-Boosting Treats

METAB-BOOSTER #1: WHITE TEA. White tea is the least processed tea and has more EGCG (epigallocatechin-3-gallate)—a mix of compounds that decrease your body's production of fat cells, according to German research.

METAB-BOOSTER #2: GRASS-FED BEEF. The conjugated linoleic acid (CLA) in grass-fed beef can boost your metabolism and help you drop belly fat, too. You'll also find CLA in dairy products from grass-fed animals (try a soft sheep's cheese, for example).

METAB-BOOSTER #3: PEANUT BUTTER FOR BREAKFAST. Eating some fat within an hour after you wake up sets your metabolism to burn fat better for the rest of the day, according to a study from the University of Alabama at Birmingham. (Don't like peanut butter? Try another healthy fat: almond or cashew butter, some macadamia nuts sprinkled on cereal or yogurt, or an avocado.)

METAB-BOOSTER #4: YOGURT. A British study found that slim people have a healthy crop of gut bacteria, which helps control how your body absorbs and metabolizes fat. Eat yogurt with live cultures to get more good bacteria, which helps your system metabolize fat faster. You'll get the same benefit from cheeses, juices, and even chocolate bars with added live cultures.

METAB-BOOSTER #5: A JUST-RIPE BANANA. Bananas that are just barely ripe are a great source of Resistant Starch—a type of carb that boosts your body's ability to burn more fat.

3 Wow Workout Benefits

You know regular physical activity is good for your heart, of course. But check out these more surprising (and pleasurable!) perks.

 IT BOOSTS YOUR MOOD. Runner's high is no myth: Regular sweat sessions up your endorphins. Many studies have found exercise even helps ease mild depression. One report in the journal *Psychosomatic Medicine* found that a group of depressed people got as much benefit from regular intense exercise as the group taking antidepressants.

 IT HIKES YOUR LIBIDO. A workout session helps keep you primed for action because it boosts your testosterone levels. It also, of course, ups your level of feel-good (and feel-frisky) endorphins. Plus, working up a sweat gets blood pumping to your nether regions, which can make you feel in the mood to hit the bedroom.

 IT HELPS YOU SLEEP. As long as you don't work out at night, exercise helps you sleep better, possibly because your stress hormones go down after you work out (they initially rise, but then fall).

TO RECAP, WORKOUTS ARE GOOD FOR...
Great mood. Hot sex. Fabulous sleep. See you at the gym!

Q. Is it safe to sit on that ledge in the steam room?

It is extremely moist and warm in a steam room. And what do bacteria love most? Warm, moist places. So it's not the optimal place to park your bare butt.

But that doesn't mean you have to live your life not enjoying any of these spa amenities. Just be smart: Put a towel, folded enough times to keep your skin away from the moisture, under your bottom. And wear underwear or a bathing suit. If you have any cuts or open sores, avoid steam rooms until healed. Wooden benches are worse than tile ones, by the way, because the cracks in the wood provide a place for germs to settle in and set up shop.

TRUE OR FALSE?

A pound of muscle weighs more than a pound of fat.

False. A pound is a pound. But muscle is denser and takes up less space than fat, so you will look sleeker at the same weight if you're building up muscle and losing fat.

• • • • • •

Q. Why do my boobs ache after running, even when I wear a good running bra?

That good bra might not be as good as you think, or it may be worn out.

You see, when we exercise, our breasts move not only up and down, according to a recent study at Oregon State University, but also side to side and forward and backward. This latter motion (backward and forward) simply isn't reined in by most sports bras.

In fact, D-cup breasts in a low-support bra can move a total of 35 inches up and down during a sweat session (a B-cup in a high-support bra barely moves an inch). That's quite a workout! That could explain your post-jog ache, huh? Solution: If you're bigger than a B-cup, choose a sports bra that has a cup for each breast. This style is way better at keeping the girls comfortably contained while you work out.

Q. I forgot my sports bra and exercised in a lacy bra—yeow! My nipples are paying the price. How can I soothe this irritation?

Oh boy, I feel your pain. This kind of hurt can be incredibly uncomfortable, and is best soothed with an old-fashioned remedy: Soak two teabags in cold water and put them directly on your nipples for 15 minutes. Repeat as often as needed. We're not exactly sure why this treatment works, though we think it has to do with the tannins in the tea. And while your raw nipples are recovering, stuff your bras with breast gel pads, which prevent your sore nipples from rubbing against bra fabric and seams; you can pick these up at maternity stores. While you're there, grab a moisturizer with lanolin ointment that's designed for sore nipples. I don't even have to tell you to always wear a fitness bra in the future, because I know you'll never make this excruciating mistake again!

• • • • • •

Q. I always have to go number two after I work out. Is something wrong with me?

Nope, what you're experiencing is perfectly normal. Exercise increases the contractions of your intestine, which propel stool along and, well, out. It also makes your food pass through your digestive tract more quickly. In fact, I often recommend at least 30 minutes a day of aerobic exercise as a natural fix for constipation.

21% of women have worn two sport bras at a time to try to control the jiggle.
Source: Health.com poll

De-Germ Your Gym Bag

Suspect you're growing stuff in there? Take a second
to get the gunk out with this quick plan.

THE BAG ITSELF We store all our icky, sweaty things in there. And we put it on the floor of the locker room, yuck. Once a week, empty your bag entirely and air it out. Wash it in the hottest water it can handle, and wipe it down with a disinfecting wipe. And going forward, don't put it on the gym bathroom floor. That's what the hook is for.

WATER BOTTLE You put your hands on every machine in the place and then use them to open your pop-top water bottle. Not so hygienic. Look for a water bottle that doesn't require you to touch the mouthpiece to drink. And if you can't give up your pop-top, simply wash it on high heat in the dishwasher after every use.

YOGA MAT It's a double-sided dirt-fest: sweat on one side and gym-floor germs on the other. And to make it worse, we roll it up still wet after we're done and leave it that way until our next class later in the week. Better plan: After class, wipe it down with a disinfecting wipe. And when you get home, unroll it so it dries completely.

WORKOUT CLOTHES We're all guilty of throwing our wet clothes into our bag and leaving them there for hours, or even overnight. The bacteria can grow and spread to your entire bag. To prevent that, keep several zip-top plastic bags in your gym bag where you can stash your damp threads. If you can't wash them right away, hang them to dry so the bacteria won't multiply.

FLIP-FLOPS They're the only barrier between you and the shower floors. Think of all that fungi! When you're finished, pop them in a plastic bag instead of putting them straight into your gym bag. When you get home, spray those bad boys with a disinfecting cleaner and let them air dry.

11: Gym Confidential

Q. My friend keeps trying to drag me to her hot yoga class, but could it be hazardous?

It could be. Bikram yoga, also known as hot yoga, takes place in a room that is 100 to 105 degrees with 40 percent humidity. Exercising in such a warm room can cause dehydration or heat stroke, so be sure to drink plenty of water (at least 16 ounces) before and during hot yoga.

Also, these conditions can be stressful on your heart, so if you have heart disease, stay away. Others who should steer clear of Bikram: children, the elderly, and pregnant women.

If you decide to give hot yoga a whirl but start to feel dizzy, faint, nauseous, or sick in any way, stop right away because you could be heading toward heat stroke. Also, if you take any prescription medication or have a serious health condition of any kind, talk to your doctor first before taking this kind of class.

Yoga is meant to be a relaxing, meditative activity, so my personal feeling is why do it in uncomfortable, potentially dangerous conditions?

• • • • • • •

Q. I'm in my 30s and still get Charley horses at night. I don't get it! I'm not a teenager.

Charley horse is a colloquial term for a painful muscle spasm of the quadriceps, leg, foot, or calf. We sometimes think of it as part of the "growing pains" many teens go through, but the fact is, you can get them at any age.

This pain can be caused by muscle strain from a workout or even tottering around in high heels. You can also get a Charley horse from dehydration or low levels of potassium or calcium. Rarely, it can be a sign of nerve injury, like a herniated disk. If it happens often, have

who knew?

Women who hate their ankles are seeing plastic surgeons to get liposuction on them (pricetag: $5,000 and up).

your doctor check your blood for calcium or potassium deficiency and do a full neurologic exam. Otherwise, try eating more foods with potassium like avocado, banana, or spinach. And be sure to warm up your muscles and cool them down with stretching before, during, and after every workout.

. . . .

Q. My crotch gets super-sweaty when I work out. It's just the grossest. What can I do?

Like your armpits, your crotch is endowed with many sweat glands. So it's normal—if not so pleasant—to be damp down below after a brisk jog or workout. Pubic hair can trap moisture, too, which can mix with bacteria and cause irritation or odor. I don't recommend you attempt to soak up sweat with a panty liner—any friction between it and you could up the odds of vaginal irritation. Instead, stick to the basics: Wear cotton undies when you work out, get a quick shower if you can, and put on fresh underwear as soon as possible.

You can defend against excess below-the-belt sweat with gym pants, shorts, and skorts made of fabrics designed to pull moisture away from your skin. Also helpful: Wear loose-fitting garments (forget about spandex) and throw all bottoms in the wash after wearing them.

HOW **BAD** IS IT *REALLY?*

To blow off showering after working out **Depends on the workout.** If you just polished off a light non-aerobic workout that didn't make you sweat, then a post-exercise shower is strictly optional. But if you're drenched at the end of your session and are sitting in damp clothes (especially damp underwear), that can lead to chafing and a rash. The dampness is also a breeding ground for bacteria or yeast, both of which can lead to infection. So don't blow off a shower after you run, bike, hit the treadmill, or do anything extreme.

Vice Advice

chapter

12

*Does what happens
in Vegas, stay in Vegas?*

12: Vice Advice

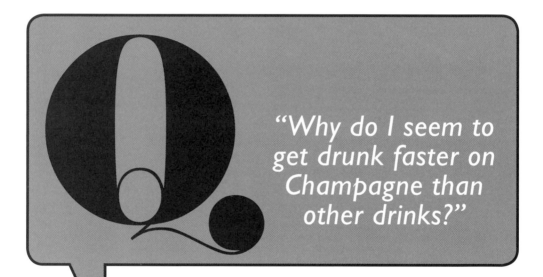

Q. *"Why do I seem to get drunk faster on Champagne than other drinks?"*

a It's not your imagination. While a glass of champagne has the same alcohol content as a glass of wine or your basic cocktail, the bubbles (gas) in champagne cause it to get absorbed faster in your stomach and into the bloodstream so you get drunk more quickly. Also, because the Champagne-making process involves two fermentations, it contains more of certain chemicals (called congeners) that make hangovers worse. Guess that's why we save the bubbly for special occasions!

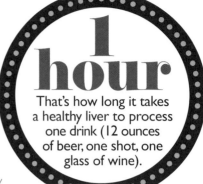

1 hour

That's how long it takes a healthy liver to process one drink (12 ounces of beer, one shot, one glass of wine).

Q. When I go out drinking and get to bed really late, I always wake up so early. Why is that?

While alcohol can make you sleepy, it actually disrupts your regular sleep patterns so that your sleep is fitful, disturbed, and, yep, shorter than usual. You're probably only sleeping a few hours, so it's more of a nap than actual sleep. If you can, take one ibuprofen and a big glass of water and try to catch another hour of zzz's.

Q. Why does beer make me pee like crazy, but wine doesn't?

Anything with alcohol in it acts as a diuretic, meaning it makes you urinate a lot. The big difference between beer and wine is the amount of liquid you're getting: With a brew, you're downing a lot more liquid. And more liquid going in means more to come out!

Q. I have friends who say, "Tequila makes me mean." Is it possible that liquor could make someone angry?

There's really nothing magical about tequila (it's not hallucinogenic, though those rumors persist). Alcohol in general depresses our inhibitions. That means we lose our usual self-control and say and do things we wouldn't normally do when sober. Some people believe we show our "true selves" when we drink too much, but all this really means is we lose our ability to rein ourselves in.

Without our usual inhibitions, some of us become very affectionate or sexual, while others may become a sad or an angry "mean drunk." Usually this behavior has nothing to do with the liquor, but is instead the bubbling up of anger that always existed but was subdued by sobriety. Just my two cents: If someone declares herself a "mean drunk" I'd take her at her word and steer clear.

* * * * * *

Q. After a night of drinking, I sometimes forget what happened at the end of the night, but it always comes back to me once my friend reminds me. That's not a blackout, right?

Well, it's a type of blackout called a fragmentary or partial blackout. That's just a fancy way to say you forgot what happened while you were drunk, but with prompting, can remember most or all of the night. It implies that you're drinking to excess and potentially putting yourself in danger.

Forgetting a tabletop dance or karaoke solo is one thing, but people who black out sometimes drive, have unprotected intercourse, spend excessive amounts of money, or engage in other high-risk behaviors. So you should take even a partial blackout as a sign that you may have a serious drinking problem that needs to be addressed.

* * * * * *

39%
of women have lied to their doctor and said they drink less than they do.
Source: Health.com poll

Q. What if I'm having full blackouts? Does that make me an alcoholic?

Not necessarily—studies of college kids show that about half of them have blacked out at some point in their lives, and they're not all problem drinkers. When you have a full blackout (called an en bloc blackout) you have zero recall, even with prompting, of a certain period of time while intoxicated.

6 Things You Should Never Lie About to Your Doctor

1) YOUR *OTHER* PILLS (HERBAL OR ALTERNATIVE MEDS).
You worry that your doc will disapprove of your Chinese herbs and megadoses of six different vitamins, so you keep it to yourself. But we really do need to know, because these remedies can react with medication—and they might even be *causing* your symptoms.

2) THE RX MEDICINES YOU TAKE. Even the ones you think have a stigma (antidepressants, sleep aids, ritalin, herpes meds). Docs don't judge patients for being on drugs (hey, we put patients on drugs!).

3) HOW SAFE YOUR SEX IS. It's tempting to give all the right answers when you're asked about your nightly habits, but if you aren't practicing safe sex (or have multiple partners at the same time who might also have multiple partners), that's vital info.

4) YOUR DIFFICULT FAMILY HISTORY. Even if it's a really sore topic (your mother's suicide, your father's alcoholism), sharing can help you avoid family weaknesses and have a happy and healthy future.

5) THAT YOU DIDN'T TAKE HER ADVICE. Sure, you may feel embarrassed to admit you didn't take the full course of medicine or blew off her low-fat diet, but if you pretend you complied, she'll assume that plan didn't work and may move on to a Plan B that's more invasive, time-consuming, or expensive.

6) ALL YOUR VICES. It can be hard to admit out loud what you do after-hours, but to truly be able to help you, your doctor needs to know if you're using recreational drugs or drinking heavily.

If you're frequently blacking out, though, you need to address your drinking as soon as possible. Blacking out puts you at risk for real immediate danger (see previous question for the risks). It also suggests you're abusing alcohol, which ups your risk of health problems down the road (liver disease, heart problems, certain cancers like ones of the throat and colon). If you don't think you can cut back on your own, ask your doctor for a referral to a substance-abuse counselor.

• • • • • • •

Q. Can too many venti lattes give me a heart attack?

If you're healthy, no. While most large studies on caffeine and heart attacks haven't found a link, a few new studies suggest that coffee can raise the risk of heart attack for people with heart disease or known risk factors for it (high blood pressure, diabetes, etc.). One study found that people most

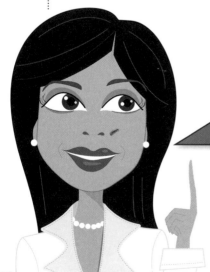

PSST, FROM DR. RAJ!
Have to tell your doctor something you think she won't want to hear (history of drug use, your fondness for one-night stands)? Take a deep breath, and just say it. See? Much better! It's out there.

in danger are those who don't normally consume a lot of caffeine (doesn't sound like you, huh?). One theory: Their hearts were less used to the temporary spike in blood pressure due to caffeine. So if you have risk factors for heart disease, you should probably avoid coffee. But if you don't, 200 to 300 milligrams of caffeine a day—about two venti lattes—shouldn't hurt you.

Caveat time: If you feel sleep-challenged, anxious, or irritable, or develop acid reflux, your body is telling you to cut back.

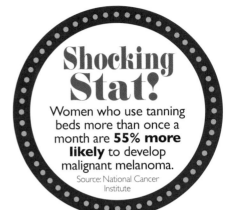

Shocking Stat!

Women who use tanning beds more than once a month are **55% more likely** to develop malignant melanoma.

Source: National Cancer Institute

• • • • • •

Q. How risky is just one visit to a tanning salon?

It's risky all right. Here's why: Skin cancer is on the rise in women under 50, and the use of tanning beds is partly to blame. While most research has examined people who visit them regularly (once a week, for example), some studies show that even a single session makes you 2.5 times more likely to get squamous cell skin cancer and 1.5 times more likely to get basal cell skin cancer, the two most common forms of the disease.

Going for a base tan before a tropical vacation might sound reasonable, but the protection this gives you is equivalent to using an SPF of 3. Not worth the risk. Instead, achieve a faux glow the safe way: Self-tanning products and cosmetic spray tans are more goof-proof than ever—and they're risk-free. Also, be sure to schedule regular skin-checks with your derm, especially if you've frequented tanning salons (or have a history of bathing under real rays). She'll be able to spy a changing mole before it becomes a bigger problem.

2 Burning Questions About Sex Addiction

 IS THERE REALLY SUCH A THING AS SEX ADDICTION—OR IT JUST A MADE-UP DISEASE TO GET CHEATERS OUT OF HOT WATER?

With notorious celebs running to sex rehab as soon as they're caught, some people may wonder if they're seeking out real treatment, or just in for a quick image-repair job. The truth is, sex addiction is real. Some therapists believe it's just a habit that becomes an obsession and compulsion; they would classify it as OCD. Others say that sex addicts are not after sex itself, but are after a dopamine (the feel-good chemical in our brains) high—and that it is in fact a chemical addiction like, say, alcoholism.

 SO DOES THAT MEAN TO FULLY RECOVER, SEX ADDICTS CAN NEVER HAVE SEX AGAIN (LIKE ALCOHOLICS CAN NEVER DRINK AGAIN)?

Well, no, abstinence isn't the end goal of sexual-addiction treatment. Doctors instead try to rehabilitate the addict to think about sex in healthier terms, to have a normal sex life with his or her partner, and to curb the urge to seek out sex anywhere and everywhere.

Q. I occasionally have a cigarette when I'm out with my friends, but none of us smokes regularly. Is it okay to just have one now and then?

It's just not. There is no safe level of smoking. Whether you're talking two packs a day or a few drags once in a blue moon, you're doing yourself harm by lighting up at all. (We also know that secondhand smoke is dangerous to non-smokers, so if you're around your friends and they're lighting up, you're upping your risk anyway.)

And so-called casual puffing actually is a dangerous slippery slope: Recent studies have shown that "social" smokers are at greater risk for heart disease and lung disease than non-smokers. In addition, they are also in danger of becoming heavier smokers over time. So once-in-a-while leads to only-on-the-weekends, and before you know it, you're up to a pack a week.

Many social smokers light up more often if alcohol is present. If that sounds like you, offer to be the designated driver and sip a diet soda or a virgin mixed drink to avoid the temptation.

• • • • • • •

Q. Is it true vodka won't give you a hangover?

Wouldn't that be nice? Sorry, the answer is no. The main reason we feel hung over is because of the effects of alcohol on our body—dehydration, low blood sugar, irritated stomach, sleep disturbance, and headache—and vodka contains alcohol so it can give you all of the above. It does, however, contain fewer congeners (chemicals that make hangovers worse), so drinking straight vodka or other lighter-colored drinks may be easier on your system than darker forms of alcohol like whiskey, brandy, or red wine. But if you have enough vodka martinis, you'll definitely feel it in the morning!

17%
of women have lied to their doctor about whether they ever smoked.
Source: Health.com poll

Past Sins

Q. I smoked a ton of pot in college but haven't touched it since. Are there any lasting effects?

We don't know all the long-term effects of marijuana, but recent studies show adults who smoked pot often as a teen have an increased risk of anxiety or depression as adults. Also, cannabis is actually worse than tobacco in terms of risk of lung cancer and lung disease, so your college pot habit means you have a higher chance of that. But you were smart to quit—your risk would have been much worse had you continued to light up.

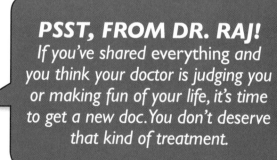

PSST, FROM DR. RAJ!
If you've shared everything and you think your doctor is judging you or making fun of your life, it's time to get a new doc. You don't deserve that kind of treatment.

Q. I smoked socially in my 20s, then quit. Should I be worried about getting lung cancer?

Congrats—quitting smoking is just about the smartest thing you could have done for your health. Your risk of smoking-related ills is related to how much you smoked and how long, so light smoking probably means your risks are minimal (certainly less than if you had continued smoking). Ten years after ditching nicotine, your risk decreases to about half of what it is for current smokers. Your risk of heart disease and stroke decrease dramatically in the first 15 years after quitting, too. So while you are at increased risk compared to someone who never lit up, that difference becomes lower and lower the longer you remain smoke-free.

Q. If it's really worrying me, should I get a lung scan?

I wouldn't if I were you. The screening of smokers and ex-smokers has not been shown to reduce death from lung cancer. And there are some significant downsides to getting a lung CT just for precautionary purposes: The test often shows nodules that turn out to be benign. That means you may have to endure biopsies and anxiety for no reason.

Plus, a CT scan will expose you to radiation, and we're just not sure yet how much that radiation scan ups your future cancer risk. So for now, just talk to your doctor and let her know your concern about your past. She'll keep an eye out for any possible lung cancer warning signs.

who knew?

Nicotine is as physically addictive as heroin.

Q. I dabbled with drugs and alcohol years ago—can that hurt my fertility now?

As long as it's all in the past, you're fine. Current drug or alcohol use, on the other hand, can definitely affect fertility by throwing off your menstrual cycles and ovulation and impairing your egg quality. And, truthfully, even drug use within one year can have an impact.

By the way, *his* sins can hurt your chances of getting pregnant, too. Drugs and alcohol can affect semen production, sperm mobility and sperm count, all of which impact fertility.

Is It Gone Yet?

Smoked or swallowed something of questionable legality? Here's how long it'll be detectable in your system.*

ALCOHOL: 6-10 hours

MARIJUANA: typically 1-2 days; up to 5 weeks for long-time habitual users

COCAINE: 1-4 days

LSD: 8 hours (it is a myth that LSD stays in your spinal cord for the rest of your life)

ECSTASY: 1-2 days

(*based on moderate use)

Q. Is it true that acid causes permanent brain damage? I'm worried because years ago I took it once!

I wouldn't worry. Some past LSD users experience occasional flashbacks—hallucinations or reliving of a "trip"—that last a few minutes and aren't permanent. Rarely, you can develop frequent distressing flashbacks or visual disturbances called Hallucinogen Persisting Perception Disorder. But if you haven't experienced either of these problems yet, you're probably okay.

In the short term, using LSD can lead to psychosis or severe depression, but those conditions happen at the time of use, not years later. Are you worried because you heard that acid stays in your system forever? Don't believe it; the drug is usually gone the next day.

· · · · · · ·

Q. How anorexic do you have to be to suffer heart damage? I starved myself constantly in my teens!

Anorexia can cause heart problems in different ways—even moderate anorexia can cause abnormal heart rhythms or even heart valve abnormalities like mitral valve prolapse. More severe starvation and weight loss can weaken heart muscle and lead to heart failure. These problems usually improve after weight is regained (although the first couple weeks of refeeding can be dangerous)—but they don't always. You're probably fine, but to ease your mind, ask your doctor for a referral to a cardiologist who will likely do an EKG and echocardiogram to check your heart's health.

TRUE OR FALSE?

When I go for my checkup, my doctor will know from my urine test if I've used drugs.

False. Urine tests can identify drugs in your system, but doctors aren't usually looking for that info in routine urine checks. Instead, they are checking for basic problems like excess protein (a sign of kidney problems), sugar (a sign of diabetes), or blood (a sign of infection, kidney stones or other kidney diseases). They don't routinely analyze urine for drugs (though they can if they want to).

On a Date

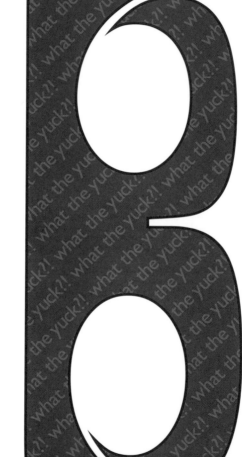

13

Boy meets girl.
Girl has soooo many
questions!

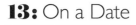

13: On a Date

Q. *"A guy I just started dating has bedbugs. Can I catch them from him?"*

a Indirectly, yes. Bedbugs, or *Cimex lectularius,* are not passed person to person—they are only attached to humans for five to ten minutes while they feed on blood (yuck, I know). The rest of the time they hide out and lay eggs in cracks and crevices on mattresses, bed frames, and sofas.

Bedbugs could jump onto your clothes or into your bag, though, and hitch a ride to your place. And these critters bite. The bites look like tiny round red spots; they're usually very itchy. Buy an anti-itch lotion (look for ones with one percent hydrocortisone) to ease the intense itchiness.

If you notice any bites, wash any potentially contaminated clothes in hot water and dry them using the hottest setting in your dryer. Or, if you can, put your contaminated clothes and belongings in a plastic bag and set them in an out-of-the-way place, like a garage, for about a week. They'll die from lack of nourishment (i.e., human blood). And call in a professional exterminator to make sure the critters are gone from your home.

· · · · · ·

WATCH WHERE YOU SLEEP

Bedbug infestations are on the rise. In New York City, there were 537 cases in 2004 and a whopping 11,000 in 2009.

Q. Do condoms *really* expire?

Yes, the latex in condoms degrades over time, making the condom a less-effective barrier to STDs or sperm. Most condoms last about five years; they'll lose their power sooner if they have spermicide. Also, they degrade more quickly in the heat or if they're bent and folded a lot, so you shouldn't store them in a back pocket or wallet. If you open a condom and it feels dry or too sticky, or if the seal is not intact, dump it.

· · · · · ·

Q. How can I stop my stomach from growling before our food arrives? So embarrassing!

Our intestines are usually moving, and even more so when we're hungry or right after we've eaten. This movement, coupled with the normal gas ever-present in your bowels, produces that telltale gurgling sound. Some people notice it more than others.

If you want to gurgle-proof your gut, eat a little something before the date (ideally, you should have small meals throughout the day anyway), and avoid foods and drinks that are notoriously gassy (soda, beans, broccoli, and chewing gum are a few big culprits).

13: On a Date

Q. Is it true if a guy smells good to you that means you're biologically compatible?

Like most things involving men and women, it's complicated! There have been several studies that showed that people are attracted to the smell of members of the opposite sex who are somewhat genetically dissimilar in terms of their immune-system genes, and are turned off by the odor of those with very similar immune-system genes. Being genetically unlike in this way has a biological advantage for the kids because theoretically they'll have both sets of genes and therefore a more diverse immune system.

But this theory has yet to be proven, and there are so many other factors that go into compatibility, I wouldn't put too much stock in this as a way to find your perfect match.

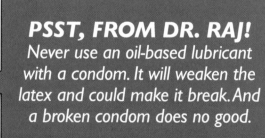

PSST, FROM DR. RAJ!
Never use an oil-based lubricant with a condom. It will weaken the latex and could make it break. And a broken condom does no good.

Q. My new guy offered me his toothbrush when I was staying over. Toothbrush sharing seems germier than kissing, but is it really?

It can be. If he is vigorously brushing his teeth, he can cause tiny abrasions in his gums. Those abrasions can bleed, so a toothbrush can harbor some nasty germs that live in the blood like hepatitis or HIV. Kissing can also expose you to someone's blood if you both have sores or cuts in your mouth. (Just fyi: For run-of-the-mill germs like those that cause a cold, they're both equally bad.) Unless you know he's been tested for everything, gargle with mouthwash instead and call it a day.

• • • • • • •

Q. Should I get the HPV vaccine?

It depends on how old you are. The human papillomavirus (HPV) vaccine prevents most of the strains of HPV that cause genital warts and cervical cancer. But it's recommended for young women 11 to 26, ideally before they become sexually active (when they haven't been exposed to HPV).

But women who are already sexually active might still benefit from the vaccine. While there's a chance you may have already been exposed to some strains of HPV, the vaccine can still protect you from other strains of HPV. It isn't FDA approved for anyone outside the 11 to 26 age group yet, but that doesn't mean you can't get vaccinated. I recommend you talk over the pros and cons with your gynecologist.

HOW **BAD** IS IT *REALLY?*
To not divulge that you have HPV

Bad. Your date can contract it from you. Most men who get HPV never have any symptoms, but you should still tell him. This STD, which is incredibly common, puts him at risk for genital warts, penile cancer, and anal cancer. Plus, he can pass it to a future partner. You'd want him to reveal any STDs he has, so you should spill, too.

13: On a Date

Q. **I get cold sores all the time. It's so embarrassing—I don't want to go on dates or even be seen at work when I have one. Is there any way to prevent them?**

Those pesky cold sores that pop up on or around your lips or nose are generally caused by a strain of the herpes simplex virus (HSV) known as HSV-1. True to the name, a cold can bring on a sore—and so can a fever, which is why they're sometimes called fever blisters. Bolstering your immune system by eating well, getting plenty of rest, and avoiding stress (that's the hard one, right?) may help you steer clear. Sun is also a common trigger, so don't ever step outside without a high-SPF lip balm.

There's no reason to suffer through embarrassing outbreaks: Ask your doctor for a prescription for an antiviral medicine. If you fill it in advance and take it at the first hint of a sore, it makes your outbreak much milder and less noticeable.

• • • • • • •

Q. **If I stay up all night, will I *still* get morning breath?**

Probably not. Saliva normally helps clear your mouth of food particles and bacteria that can cause an odor. When we sleep, we don't produce as much saliva as when we are awake, and the resulting dry mouth is what causes bad breath.

If you stay up all night, your body will continue to pump out saliva, and you shouldn't get morning breath—or at least not as bad as you would if you dozed. To ease that post-sleep stench, brush and floss well and drink a glass of water before bed.

41% of women have been too embarrassed to ask a sexual partner if he had an STD.

Source: Health.com poll

Q. I'm afraid I'm a loud snorer. Is there anything I can do to prevent this from happening when I spend the night with my new man?

You mean aside from lying awake all night? First, don't drink alcohol. It can make snoring worse by relaxing your throat's muscles. When you breathe in and out, those relaxed muscles vibrate, and you snore.

Also, congested nasal passages contribute to snoring, so you might want to bring along a box of nasal strips and pop one on before climbing in bed (just say you have allergies). They may not be pretty, but they open up your nasal passages from the outside in, letting air flow more easily.

If these moves don't help you get your snoring under control, you may have obstructive sleep apnea—a serious respiratory condition—and should make an appointment to discuss this problem with your doctor.

But, to be honest, you shouldn't be embarrassed about this or any other bodily function. If this is going to be a long-term relationship, sooner or later he's going to hear you snore. And if he dumps you because of that, what a jerk!

TRUE OR FALSE?

The size of his foot (or finger… or nose…) predicts the size of his you-know-what.

False. Though many a woman has looked from her date's feet to his groin, there's absolutely no predicting the size of his package, according to a study published in the *British Journal of Urology International*. In fact, you can't tell his size by looking at any body part except *that* part. Aren't you glad we cleared that one up?

Fashion Forward

chapter

14

*When skinny
jeans attack*

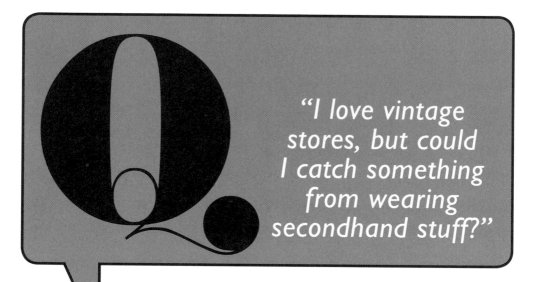

> *"I love vintage stores, but could I catch something from wearing secondhand stuff?"*

Heard of scabies? The most common stowaways in secondhand threads are *Sarcoptes scabiei* (aka scabies)—eight-legged mites that burrow into your skin and cause intense itching and blisters.

BUT YOU CAN STILL LOOK FABULOUS IN VINTAGE WITH THESE TIPS:

Be picky about your stores. Good vintage and consignment shops (as opposed to the rummage sale in a church basement) are careful about what goods they take, so you're less likely to have a problem.

Bag your buys. Before you wear someone else's cast-offs, starve the mites. Keep all your purchases in a plastic bag and stash them in the garage or basement for two weeks. They'll die of starvation.

Wash clothes well. Take the bag of retro threads straight to your laundry room. Don't risk someone opening the bag and spreading the possible mites around. Wash in hot water and dry them on high heat. If something can't be washed at home, take it to a dry cleaner.

Check out your bites. If you've already developed an itch and blisters, it's time to see your doctor. She may prescribe permethrin or crotamiton, topical meds that kill the bugs quickly (though you may still itch for several weeks). And because scabies is contagious (the mites are easy to pass around), your doctor will likely treat everyone in your family and others you all come into close contact with on a regular basis, even if they don't show any signs of scabies yet.

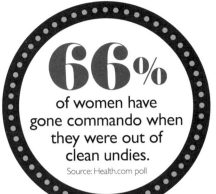

66% of women have gone commando when they were out of clean undies.

Source: Health.com poll

Q. Sometimes I'll wear my jeans several times before washing them. Is that sanitary?

So you've got a pair you love above all others? No worries: As long as you're wearing underwear, this is fine. But on the off chance you're going commando, you should wash your jeans before slipping them back on. Here's why: There's a slight risk of bacteria growing on your denim, which could give you an infection.

Q. When bathing suit shopping, how could that paper crotch guard that *everyone* touches possibly protect me from catching something nasty?

You're on to something here: It can't. The paper just protects the garment from getting stained. It doesn't protect you from nasty infections or pubic lice. So you must always wear your underwear when trying on a bathing suit—it's lumpy, yes, but necessary. And once you find your perfect suit, wash it in warm or even hot water before wearing it.

Q. What's the worst thing you can catch from your thong?

In theory, since your thong is just touching *your* body, you won't catch anything you don't already have. In fact, studies have never been able to find a link between thongs and infections. But some women do notice an increase in UTIs and yeast infections when they wear these undies, so you'll have to decide if it's worth the risk to avoid visible panty lines.

The potential problem with these undergarments is that fecal bacteria can move more easily from the rectum to your vagina, and then work their way into your urinary tract, possibly causing a UTI. Also, tight thongs may irritate the vagina and surrounding skin, which opens you up to infection.

No need to switch to granny panties: Just use basic common sense—meaning, good hygiene. Don't wear the same thong for more than a day, and wear them for limited periods of time. If you start to notice any itching or irritation on your outer skin, switch to a loose cotton pair of undies instead. And if you develop a UTI or yeast infection, don't wear a thong until the infection is history.

PSST, FROM DR. RAJ!
We really and truly don't care what bra and underwear you wear to office visits. But if it will make you uncomfortable to have your doc see your laciest thong, wear a more basic pair. Your choice!

When Good Feet Go Bad

Got shoe-related foot problems? Here's your primer
so you can decode the lumps, bumps, and pain:

PUMP BUMP

What it is: An enlargement of the bone in the back of your heel.

Why you get it: As you walk, shoes irritate the back of your heel, causing painful inflammation and swelling in the bursa, a fluid-filled sac between the tendon and bone.

How it is treated: Anti-inflammatory medicines might reduce the swelling in the bursa. Your doctor might also suggest a cortisone shot—or even surgery to remove the excess bone growth.

MORTON'S NEUROMA

What it is: An abnormal growth of nerve tissue between the third and fourth toe that can cause pain and burning in the toes and foot.

Why you get it: It might develop as a response to pressure or irritation of the toes caused by high heels or high-impact stress like running.

How it is treated: Avoid wearing too-tight or pointy-toed shoes so you won't cause any more pressure. Special pads spread the toes to keep them from squeezing the nerve. If these don't work, your doctor may recommend surgery.

HAMMERTOE

What it is: A condition that occurs when toes bend up at the joint (from the side, the toe resembles an upside-down V). Common in the second through fifth toes.

Why you get it: You may be genetically predisposed to this problem and can't help but develop it. If you're squeezing your feet into shoes with narrow toes, you might be causing the problem.

How it is treated: It can sometimes be treated by changing shoes (away from the pointy toes) or using inserts to take pressure off the toe.

BLISTER

What it is: A pocket of raised skin filled with fluid.

Why you get it: The skin is irritated due to friction, and the top layer of skin separates and fills with fluid. A blister usually develops from poor-fitting or too-tight shoes.

How it is treated: Don't pop the blister because it's more prone to infection if open. The fluid will eventually recede. Until the blister and irritation are gone, cover the sensitive spot with an adhesive bandage or gauze.

Decode Your Shoes

You don't have to trade your Manolo Blahniks for Birkenstocks any time soon, but you should know what your favorite pairs are doing to your body. Here's the rundown:

STILETTOS are bad for your feet, knees, and back. They apply uneven pressure to all your joints and can be painful in the short term and cause problems like pump bumps or bunions in the future. You also risk twisting an ankle (only so many people can balance in 4-inch heels). If you have to wear them, keep it to a minimum—less than three hours at a time.

WEDGES are better for your feet than stilettos because they provide a bit more support than the stiletto—your weight is on the ball of your feet in stilettos—but they're still not great. If you have knee problems or arthritis in your knees, avoid the wedge.

MULES give you zero ankle support. You risk rolling your ankle when you walk in these. They can also cause toe and upper-foot pain.

FLIP-FLOPS are—surprise!—almost as bad as stilettos. You've got no arch or ankle support, and when you walk, you have to crunch up your toes to keep the shoe on. That might mean toe, heel, or foot cramps. They're okay for short-term use, but don't make them your go-to shoe.

BALLET FLATS give you no support. They're almost a glorified slipper. You also up your chances of developing plantar fasciitis, inflammation of the tissue in your heel.

SO WHAT'S A "DO!" SHOE? One with cushioning, support, and gobs of room for your toes. And for everyday use, try to keep the heel below one inch (nights out are a different story!).

Q. I have developed ugly, painful bunions. Do I have to stop wearing my high heels?

Not necessarily, but you should skip the narrow-toe shoes. Most bunions are inherited, but narrow shoes with a small toe box can sometimes cause them. Bunions form when bone grows abnormally at the base of the big toe in the joint between your toe and foot. As they develop, they turn the big toe inward toward the smaller toes, and the enlarged joint can become inflamed, red, and painful. Women tend to have more trouble with bunions than men, thanks in part to our love affair with tough-on-the-tootsies footwear. A recent study said most of us wear shoes a size too small!

Make sure any style you wear provides at least half an inch of space between the end of your longest toe and the shoe tip. The shoe should conform to the shape of your foot and be comfortable across the widest part. How you walk could also be part of the problem: Placing too much stress on the big toe or the inside of your foot can cause bunions, along with a host of other problems, like back pain.

If your bunions hurt, see a podiatrist: She may suggest special padding to stop the irritation and abrasion and/or anti-inflammatory medication or cortisone injections to reduce the swelling and pain. Orthotic shoes or inserts may also help by keeping your feet in the ideal position as you walk.

TRUE OR FALSE?

You can get a sunburn right through your shirt

True. Thin clothing does not protect you from UV rays, especially if you're wet. If you are prone to burning or will be outside for long hours in the sun, wear special sun-protective clothing. It has SPF in the fibers, just like sunscreen. Don't have that? Wear fabrics that have a tight weave.

Q. How tight would jeans have to be to cause internal damage?

In general, tight jeans can lead to health annoyances, but not *damage*. Too-snug denim can cause vaginal irritation and may put pressure on the bladder, which could bring on a UTI. Form-fitting blues could also rub your skin and cause an uncomfortable irritation or inflammation. Beyond that, very tight jeans can affect your intestine's ability to expand and contract normally (like with eating or drinking). That can be very uncomfortable as well, but it probably won't lead to permanent damage.

Strange but true: There have been cases of tingling and numbness when nerves are trapped or cut off because of tight jeans. This is known as Tingling Thigh Syndrome—a compression of the lateral femoral cutaneous nerve, which runs across the outside of your thigh. High heels might make it worse because they throw the pelvis forward, compressing the nerve even more. But this is incredibly rare.

Bottom line: Your clothes shouldn't cause you pain. If your jeans do, buy a bigger pair. Or try "jeggings," comfy leggings disguised as skinny jeans.

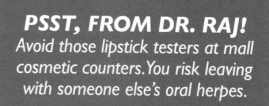

PSST, FROM DR. RAJ!
Avoid those lipstick testers at mall cosmetic counters. You risk leaving with someone else's oral herpes.

De-Germ Your Makeup Bag

It can be hard to part ways with your favorite compacts and tubes, but if you hang on to beauty products too long they can grow nasty bacteria, which then get transferred onto your face. Keep your beauty stash safe with these strategies:

MASCARA

Average life span: four to six months
Swap out your mascara every four to six months or as soon as it starts smelling funky and depositing more clumps than color. Take no chances with eye products—germ-ridden formulas can cause infections and sties. Toss your wand if you have an eye infection.

FOUNDATION

Average life span: one year
Most formulas—liquids, creams, and compacts—can last up to a year if kept out of direct sunlight and away from heaters. But once your liquid starts to separate, your cream thickens, or your compact color develops a rubbery aroma, it's time to toss it.

CONCEALER

Average life span: one year
If you use a pan or stick formula, you'll know it's gone bad when it cracks or turns tough and elastic-like. It's time to throw out your liquid concealer if it separates, appears oily, and/or smells rancid.

BLUSH AND EYE SHADOW

Average life span: one to two years
Expect creams to last one year, powders about two. If your powder grows a white crust or starts to crumble before that time, chuck it.

LIPSTICK

Average life span: eight months
Unless it turns gooey, smells rubbery, or no longer applies color to your lips, you can safely use lipstick for at least eight months. Of course, if your lipstick tube comes into contact with a cold sore or another type of infection, kiss it goodbye.

MAKEUP BRUSHES

Average life span: a year or longer
Natural-hair brushes can last almost a lifetime, if taken care of. Wash them once a week with gentle soap and warm water, and then set them on a table to dry with the brush end hanging off the edge. Synthetic brushes, used for creams, last only about a year and need to be cleaned twice a week with an alcohol-based cleaner.

14: Fashion Forward

Q. I'm thinking about getting my nose pierced. Is this dangerous—or reversible?

Most people won't have any problems. But whenever a needle meets skin, there are some risks, mostly slight: bleeding, allergic reaction to the jewelry (it should be made of silver or gold, though many people can tolerate stainless steel), and nerve damage in and around the piercing site. There's also a small risk of contracting a serious infection, like hepatitis C.

You'd be wise to have your piercing done in an establishment that's licensed by your state or local government. But do your own due diligence, too: The facilities should be sparkling clean. The technician should use a sterile needle, not a piercing gun, wash his or her hands, and don gloves before doing the job. (Try to observe some work in progress before you sit down for your own.) You should be given detailed instructions on keeping the piercing clean, as well as an antibiotic cleanser. While the spot is healing, wash your hands before touching it.

If you decide later that you don't like the piercing, most holes will close up over time once you stop wearing jewelry, although there may be a small scar.

· · · · · · ·

Q. Wearing heavy pierced earrings has totally stretched out my holes, and they look so ugly. Is it true I can get that fixed?

Yes. An ear, nose, and throat (ENT) doctor or plastic surgeon can perform a relatively simple procedure to repair those holes. They will place a few sutures in the ear to close most of the stretched-out hole—they're literally sewing it up. Or they can sew up the hole completely and create a new one nearby.

Injectable fillers like Restylane can also be used to fill in the stretched-out skin. But if you get this procedure done, avoid heavy earrings for a long time. Otherwise, you'll just stretch the holes right back out, and it might be more difficult to fix next time.

Q. I stayed over at a girlfriend's last night but forgot underwear. She offered me a pair. They're clean, but is that gross? Could I catch something?

It's not likely. If they're clean, basically anything you could catch (such as an STD) should be killed before you get your hands on them. They should have gone through a hot-water wash and high-heat dry cycle to zap all the germs. But, since you can't be completely sure how diligently your friend washes her clothes, you might turn them down. Personally, I would turn mine inside out or go commando rather than risk getting something from borrowed undies.

0%

The increase in your risk of breast cancer if you wear an underwire bra.

· · · · · · ·

Q. Help, my gold ring is turning my finger green! Is this something I should be worried about?

Were you a princess in a former life? Your skin is reacting to the fact that the ring isn't pure gold but contains a filler metal, such as copper. Some of us turn green from copper, others don't. It's harmless for the most part, but if you continue to wear that bauble, the stain could actually become permanent.

A lot of gold jewelry that is less than than 15-carat gold has some copper mixed in, so stick to 18-carat gold, platinum, stainless steel, or titanium. If you're really attached to that particular ring, just paint a layer of clear nail polish on the part of the ring that touches your finger.

The Men's Room

chapter

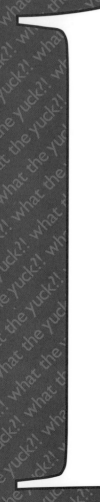

What's up with his body?

15: The Men's Room

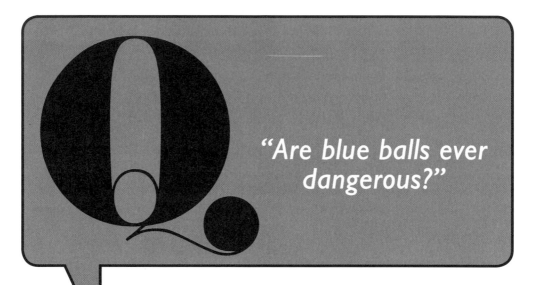

Q. *"Are blue balls ever dangerous?"*

a No—though you'd never know it by all the griping! Pelvic vasocongestion (the technical name for what guys call blue balls) occurs when a man is sexually aroused for a long period of time without release, aka orgasm. Here's what happens: During arousal, blood flow increases to the penis and testicles—they swell and sometimes have a bluish tint (perhaps that's where the name comes from). The buildup of blood can sometimes cause an aching feeling if the guy isn't able to ejaculate. It's not dangerous, and it will go away on its own within 15 minutes once the arousal has ceased. Sorry, guys, no sympathy on this one.

Q. Why do some normal-weight guys have breasts?

Gynecomastia—or enlarged breast tissue in men—is caused by an imbalance of estrogen and testosterone. All men produce small amounts of estrogen and larger amounts of testosterone (the opposite is true for women). If the amount of estrogen increases or the amount of testosterone decreases, the breast tissue could swell or grow, creating breasts.

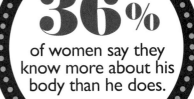

36% of women say they know more about his body than he does.

Source: Health.com poll

Age can be one factor. A hormonal imbalance can occur spontaneously during puberty or as a man ages. In fact, most men with gynecomastia are between 50 and 80. In the case of pubescent teenagers, the hormones usually balance out, and the breast size will return to normal within a year.

Medicines, like antidepressants, anti-ulcer meds, and prostate and heart meds can also cause this condition. Other culprits include alcohol, marijuana, or anabolic steroids.

Several health conditions can also cause men to develop breasts. These include hyperthyroidism, liver or kidney failure, and tumors, especially those on the adrenal or pituitary glands.

This is usually a very sensitive subject with guys. Between the shame they feel and the ridicule they get from others, it's often hard for them to seek out help. But a good doctor should be able to pinpoint the cause and treat it through lifestyle changes or medications to control the hormones. In rare cases, the excess breast tissue doesn't respond to treatment, but if the guy wants to, he can have it removed surgically.

Q. Why do I get more bug bites than my husband? Do mosquitoes like women more?

What can I say? We are just sweeter! But in all seriousness, we only know of one group that definitely attracts more mosquitoes than the rest of the population: women with buns in the oven. Moms-to-be exhale more carbon dioxide, which attracts mosquitoes. Women who wear perfumes or beauty products that contain a lot of fragrance also tend to appeal to nibbling insects. So if you get dozens of bites in one night while your man gets just one, it may be because your personal care products are more attractive to the bugs.

Another possibility: It only seems like you're getting more bites because you react more to the bites. Some people get major redness, swelling, and itchiness while others don't react at all.

To protect yourself, apply an insect repellant before going out; most of them really do work well. If you're particularly bite-prone or just don't want to end up as dinner for the mosquitoes, wear long sleeves and long pants in addition to bug repellant. And avoid sweet-smelling lotions, perfumes, and body washes if you know you're going to be spending the day outdoors. Hopefully that'll cut down on the biting.

• • • • • •

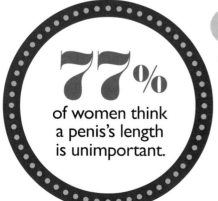

77% of women think a penis's length is unimportant.

Q. Is it true that only guys are color blind?

Nope. Color blindness is usually a genetically-determined condition (it's inherited), and while it does happen in men ten times more often than it does in women, we can be color blind, too.

Q. Why do guys burp and fart so much? It's almost like they like to do it!

Surprisingly, there is no difference in the amount of gas expelled by men and women (either through burping or flatulence). Shocking, I know! We women are just trained from a young age to be more discreet about our emissions than men. They let it rip, and we sneak off to another room.

• • • • • •

Q. Is it true laptops can make my guy infertile?

It's possible—at least in the short term. Studies have shown that resting laptops on the lap can raise scrotal temperature, thanks to a combo of the heat of the computer and the fact that men keep their knees tight together to hold the laptop in place. And an elevated scrotal temp can kill sperm, which is why couples who are trying to conceive are often told that the guy should avoid hot tubs and switch from briefs to boxers.

Whether laptop use affects long-term fertility has not been proven, but it's a good idea for your man to avoid putting his laptop directly on his lap if you are trying to conceive. Place some sort of barrier, even a book, between the computer and his lap.

TRUE OR FALSE?

His penis can break during rough-ish sex. **True.** Penis fractures, while very rare, do happen. They can be caused by his erect penis hitting something hard—like your pubic bone, for example. They can also happen if he gets carried away and mistakenly plunges in the wrong direction. Of course, there aren't any bones in the penis to break, but the covering of the corpora cavernosa— the tissues inside the penis that fill with blood during an erection—can tear or rupture. This causes extreme pain and can result in a bent penis. Surgery is sometimes necessary to fix it. If your guy experiences unbearable pain during or after sex, or there's obvious damage to the penis, head to the ER ASAP.

15: The Men's Room

HOW **BAD** IS IT *REALLY?*

For my guy to take a Viagra so we can have a marathon sex session. **So SO bad.** If your guy doesn't have erectile dysfunction, he shouldn't be messing with Viagra. He could seriously damage his heart, and, of course, his penis. He might also experience dizziness and blurry vision, and in some people Viagra causes blood pressure to bottom out, which can make him faint. For your guy's sake, don't let him do this.

Q. Why do some men have premature ejaculation?

There are many psychological and biological factors that can play a role in premature ejaculation. Is this a new relationship? He might be overthinking how to please you and so worried about maintaining an erection that he finishes more quickly than he was anticipating.

Other possible causes for the rockets taking off too soon: relationship problems (the troubles can affect his self-esteem); feeling rushed (like when you're going for a quickie—just not that quick); hormonal imbalances; abnormal levels of the brain chemicals called neurotransmitters; and even a medical issue like an inflamed prostate.

Of course, sometimes finishing early just means that he finished early. It happens to most guys every now and then. Rest a second and go again.

If your guy is quick to finish, try not to make him feel ashamed about it; that will only make the situation worse. But if it's happening a lot, you may want to bring it up in a supportive way and encourage him to talk to his doctor. There are treatments ranging from anesthetic creams to sex therapy that may just help him last longer.

· · · · · · ·

Q. Why does my guy always wake up with an erection?

Take this as a good sign—all his parts are in good working order. Most men experience three to five erections during REM sleep; this is known as nocturnal penile tumescence. So it's highly likely that a guy will wake up with one—and often.

In fact, if your guy is having erectile problems and goes to see a doctor, one of the first questions the doc will ask him is: Are you still getting morning erections? If he is, it means his problem isn't physical, and they'll know to look elsewhere.

Get Him to Give A Hoot About His Health

So your guy avoids the doctor—as well as gyms and green veggies? Here's how to (nicely) nudge him in the right direction.

 APPEAL TO HIS VANITY. If he doesn't want to lose weight or seems less-than-thrilled about the idea of working out, tell him how hot he looks when he's jogging next to you.

 GIVE IT A PURPOSE. Remind him that you want and need him to be around.

 JUST DO IT. Sometimes the hardest thing is just making the appointment, so make it for him. Once it's booked, he can't say he forgot to call. You already did that.

 GO WITH HIM. It might be easier for him to be honest and talk about his health if you're with him, even if you don't say a word.

 BE A GOOD EXAMPLE. If you're pushing him to exercise but sitting on the sofa yourself, I bet your advice is falling on deaf ears. Instead, get up and hit the gym together. You can also have fun cooking healthy as a team.

 AND WHATEVER YOU DO: DON'T PUSH TOO HARD. You may just push him in the other direction, and you definitely don't want that.

Q. Am I more likely to catch an STD from an uncircumcised guy?

As you may have heard, there has been quite a bit of controversy surrounding this subject in recent years. Studies do suggest that men who are uncircumcised are more likely to contract STDs, including HIV, herpes, HPV, and syphilis, and therefore are more likely to pass them on to you.

But here's my take: When you have sex with a new partner, always use a condom, whether he's circumcised or not. And remember, the only way to know for sure if he has an STD or not is to have him get tested.

• • • • • • •

Q. Why does he lose hair on his head and grow it in his ears?

Male pattern baldness, which is the most common type of hair loss in men, usually starts with hair loss on the top of the head and progresses to complete baldness. But for some reason, ear, chest, and back hair are usually spared while the head's hair jumps ship. And we don't know exactly why ear and nose hair seems to grow thicker and longer just as hair up top is thinning—one theory is that the hormone dihydrotestosterone, or DHT for short, which causes baldness, prompts ear and nose hair to grow more.

who knew?

Most men have one testicle that is larger or hangs lower than the other. In fact, 62% of men say their right testicle is the larger one.

Q. My new man has only one testicle. Does that mean he's infertile?

Probably not. The other testicle still is capable of producing millions of sperm—which is more than enough to get you pregnant—and should pump out enough testosterone for him to have a normal sex drive. (It's like women who have only one ovary—in most cases, it can still get the job done.)

However, if at some point you decide to have a baby together, you might want to find out *why* he has one testicle. Some conditions, like testicular cancer or epididymitis, result in the loss of one testicle and the dysfunction of the other leading to infertility. But these problems are unusual.

· · · · · ·

Q. Why do guys get "shrinkage" in water?

Exposure to cold water (or cold air) causes the blood vessels in the penis and testicles to clamp down, resulting in less blood flow to the area—and less blood flow means shrinkage. The penis and testicles also draw closer to the body to keep warm, making them appear smaller. It's only temporary, though—as you probably know, everything returns to full size when the temperature returns to normal.

HOW MUCH DO GUYS REALLY THINK ABOUT SEX?

It's not every seven seconds, like you may have heard, but it's more than we do: 54% of men think about sex at least every day, compared with only 19% of women who think about it daily, according to research from the University of Chicago.

4 Signs You Should Take Him to the ER

 HE HAS THE "WORST HEADACHE OF HIS LIFE." He may have an undiagnosed brain aneurysm or other potentially life-threatening condition and needs to go the emergency room pronto.

 HE HAS STROKE SYMPTOMS. An easy way to remember the symptoms is FAST:

F: Check for numbness or weakness on his Face by asking him to smile. If one side droops or isn't able to smile, it might be a stroke.

A: Ask him to raise his Arms. If he can't raise one arm or one arm drifts down, it may be a stroke.

S: If his Speech is slurred or hard to understand, it could be a sign of a stroke. Ask him to repeat a simple sentence.

T: The key to surviving a stroke is Time. If you recognize the symptoms of stroke, call 911 or get to a hospital quickly.

 HE HAS UNEXPLAINED CHEST PAIN OR SHORTNESS OF BREATH. He may describe it as tightness in his chest. It may come and go but will usually last for several minutes. This can be a sign of a heart attack. Don't let him keep saying, "It'll go away." It might not, so get him to the hospital.

 HE PASSES OUT. If he loses consciousness, don't wait to see how he is when he wakes up—call 911 immediately.

Q. Why are guys always adjusting their package? We don't scratch our privates in public!

In this situation, we women have it better: Our privates aren't hanging out and flapping around. And to be honest, if we had three things hanging in our underwear (two testicles and a penis) and our underwear barely gave them any support, we would probably be adjusting a lot too.

Guys can get chafing or itching in that area easily, especially in summer weather, when everything gets a little sticky and sweaty. The testicles can also become twisted or caught in their underwear. Personally I'd rather see them make a quick adjustment than try to slyly dance their balls into a better position.

Is he normal?

The average erect penis measures 5 to 7 inches in length and 1.25 to 1.6 inches in diameter.

• • • • • • •

Q. If my boyfriend smokes, is that dangerous to me?

Absolutely. Secondhand smoke increases your risk of all of the same diseases smoking does: cancer, emphysema, heart disease. And breathing in someone else's smoke is even more harmful for children than adults—so just imagine the consequences if you end up marrying this smoker.

Life 3.0

chapter

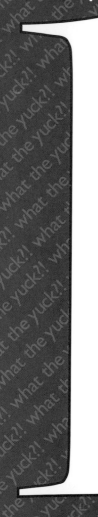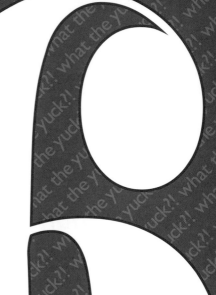

How do you avoid iPad neck? BlackBerry thumb? Download the answers here.

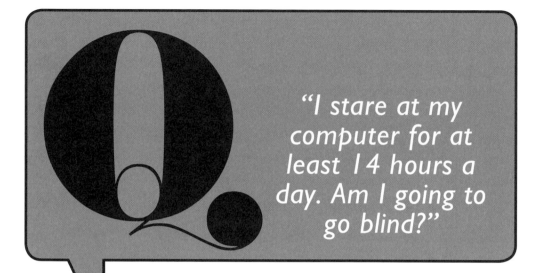

"I stare at my computer for at least 14 hours a day. Am I going to go blind?"

Staring at a computer screen can certainly cause eyestrain and fatigue, but you won't go blind. Instead, your eyes may feel tired or you may get eye pain or headaches. And of course, squinting may lead to wrinkles.

There are a few things you can do to help your eyes out. Look away from your computer screen every 20 minutes or so to give your eyes a break. Just glance outside or down the hall for about 20 seconds; repeat that move throughout the day.

To minimize eye and neck pain, position your computer screen so it's slightly below eye level; the ideal distance between you and the screen is 20 to 28 inches. At that position, you shouldn't have to lean forward or strain your neck to see the screen. Adjust the location or angle of your computer screen so that there isn't any glare, or get an anti-glare filter. Glare on a screen makes your eyes have to work even harder.

Of course, it's important to see your eye doctor once a year to check for changes in your eyesight and update your glasses and contacts accordingly. Depending on your needs, he might even prescribe some reading glasses to use, particularly when you're working on the computer.

• • • • • •

Q. How germy is the average iPhone? Everyone's always touching mine!

Very—and you just identified why. Lots of people touch it! Also, you have touched (or other people have touched) tons of surfaces before getting your hands on your phone—doorknobs, elevator buttons, toilet handles. Yuck! Keep antibacterial wipes handy to wipe it down periodically (and more often during germy times of the year like flu season). And be picky: Limit the number of people you allow to play with your phone.

• • • • • •

Q. I have to travel a lot for my new job. Will I get sick more often if I'm a frequent flyer?

That's a good question—more and more of us worry about coming down with something from the recycled air on planes. But actually, that air is probably better for you than most air in office buildings. It's well filtered before it's blown back out, so it shouldn't make you sick.

However, being in a closed cabin with all those other passengers (some of whom may be sick without showing symptoms yet) can increase your chances of catching a cold, flu virus, or some other nasty bug. And it's not just the others on your flight you have to worry about: Previous fliers might have left behind more than a completely-filled-in Sudoku—namely, germs—on the seat, seatbelt, magazines, headrest, or overhead bin.

700%
The increase in the amount of time spent on Facebook from April 2008 to April 2009.

That's why it's a good idea to bring antibacterial gel with you (in a container smaller than 3 ounces, of course) and even some antibacterial wipes (for wiping down your seat). Use the gel frequently while traveling, and especially before eating.

* * * * * *

Q. I carry everything in my handbag and it weighs a ton. Can I get stooped over to one side from it?

Yes, you can: Carrying a heavy purse on one shoulder can trigger shoulder and back pain. It can cause posture issues as well—usually because you are compensating for the weight by hunching one shoulder. That causes a postural imbalance, and after years and years, it might be very visible.

It's best to limit the weight of your bag to three pounds, and for heavier loads use backpacks or roller bags. Not the most fashionable, I know, but it's a choice between being fashionable and having back pain.

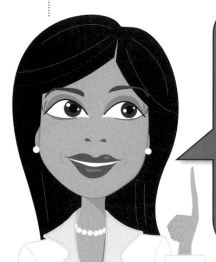

PSST, FROM DR. RAJ!
Many traditional doctors are unfamiliar with alternative medicine or have legitimate safety concerns about it. If you're a strong believer in alternative medicine, make that clear. And if your doc isn't open to it, you may want to find an MD that practices integrative medicine or incorporates alt med into her practice.

Q. I live on my cell phone—am I going to get brain cancer?

To be honest, the jury is still out on this. Recently, a prominent neuroscientist caused a ruckus by sending out an email to his colleagues advising them to limit their cell phone use because he believes it increases the risk of brain tumors. But, so far, studies just don't back him up.

A 30-year study on the incidence of brain tumors in Scandinavia found no increase in tumors even after cell phones became more popular. If there was a connection, we would have expected to see an increase in tumors in the last few years of the study, but that didn't happen.

But until we know more, using a cell phone in moderation is a good idea, especially for children, whose developing brains are more susceptible to radiation effects. Have to chat? Use a speaker phone or a headset to keep the phone from being pressed right up to your head. And while you're at it, don't carry your phone in a pocket (meaning pressed up against your body), either.

• • • • • • •

HOW **BAD** IS IT *REALLY?*

To go through those full-body scanners at the airport

Not so bad. According to the TSA, the radiation emitted by the machine is 10,000 times less powerful than a cell phone, so if you're a leisure or infrequent traveler, you have nothing to worry about. If you're traveling multiple times a week or if you just don't want to use the scanners, you can always request a hand search. It'll take more time, but you won't have to risk any radiation.

Q. Can I catch H1N1 flu from my cat?

Probably not. Cats can contract other influenzas such as avian flu (by eating an infected bird, for example), but we haven't seen any cases of cats giving the flu to humans. Honestly, if your cat does get H1N1, odds are she caught it from you.

Still, if your cat is sick during flu season, it doesn't hurt to play it safe. Get her checked out by a vet, and wash your hands any time you touch her.

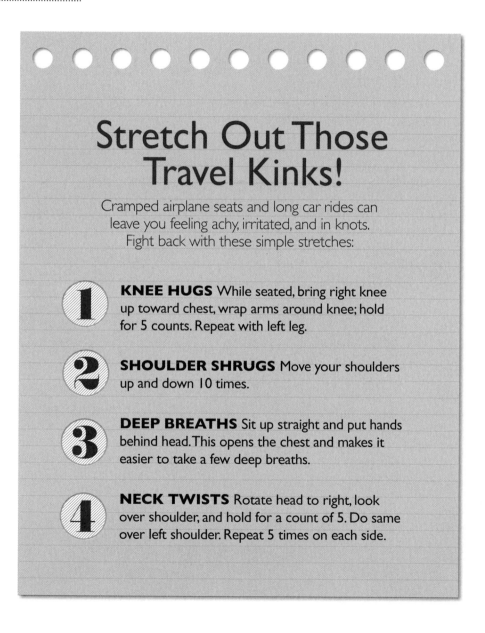

Stretch Out Those Travel Kinks!

Cramped airplane seats and long car rides can leave you feeling achy, irritated, and in knots. Fight back with these simple stretches:

1 **KNEE HUGS** While seated, bring right knee up toward chest, wrap arms around knee; hold for 5 counts. Repeat with left leg.

2 **SHOULDER SHRUGS** Move your shoulders up and down 10 times.

3 **DEEP BREATHS** Sit up straight and put hands behind head. This opens the chest and makes it easier to take a few deep breaths.

4 **NECK TWISTS** Rotate head to right, look over shoulder, and hold for a count of 5. Do same over left shoulder. Repeat 5 times on each side.

Q. Can you get trustworthy health information online?

First a caveat: Reading even good medical web sites may put you in an unnecessary panic, or falsely reassure you. There's no substitute for an actual doctor's visit.

That said, you can find good advice online. I trust information from academic medical centers, such as New York University (www.med.nyu.edu) and the Mayo Clinic (www.mayoclinic.com). I also trust the Centers for Disease Control and Prevention (www.cdc.gov). Many large consumer health web sites, such as our own Health.com and Web MD, provide carefully vetted information, too. Just be wary of any site that's trying to sell you something (supplements, etc).

• • • • • •

Q. My laptop is always on my lap. Am I blasting my ovaries with radiation?

No, there's no radiation risk. Computers are vastly improved from a few decades ago (when radiation was a problem). However, some laptops can get very hot when used for a while—sometimes so hot they can burn your skin slightly. It's a good idea to use a thick cushion, lap desk, or table rather than keep your computer directly on your lap.

TRUE OR FALSE?

It's safe to store your medical records online. **True, if you're smart about it.** Electronic personal health records offer a lot of benefits. By having your whole medical history (including allergies, immunizations, medications, and test results) in one place, you can easily keep your doctors updated on your info and help them coordinate care with specialists. If you get sick while you're traveling, you or your physicians can access the information from anywhere. But how do you ensure the info is safe? Whether you use a web-based tool or a portable format like USB, make sure it requires a password to access it, and you read and understand the privacy and security policies *before* storing your info.

Q. I find I'm listening to my iPod at higher volumes lately—does that mean I'm going deaf?

It could. Audiologists and hearing experts have been sounding the alarm over hearing loss associated with MP3 players for a few years now. Twenty-six million adults have high-frequency hearing loss caused by exposure to loud noises—aka noise-induced hearing loss (NIHL).

The risk of hearing loss from an iPod depends on how loud you're cranking it. Most iPods have a maximum decibel level (decibels are how we measure sound) of 100, but a few independent studies have found they can go as high as 120.

So what does that mean? Well, the sound of an ambulance siren is about 120 decibels. Would you listen to that for several hours every day of the week? (The average American who has an iPod listens to her iPod two hours every day.) Here's another way to think about it: By law, employees exposed to on-the-job noise above 115 decibels for longer than 15 minutes must have sound-protection equipment.

You might be saying to yourself, "Well, I only listen to it halfway up most of the time." That's good; it's possible you're not getting yours high enough to cause any damage (sounds below 75 decibels don't usually harm hearing). But hearing loss can be the result of a one-time exposure to an intense sound, or repeated exposure to sounds at or above 85 decibels. The louder the noise, the shorter time period before NIHL begins.

Have you ever turned your iPod up to rock out to your favorite Nirvana song? Or pumped up the volume to drown out background street noises? You may have permanently damaged your hearing.

To prevent further harm, always use the middle setting or lower on your iPod's volume control. As a rule of thumb, if you are using earphones and someone next to you can hear your music (or worse—identify the song!), it's too loud.

73%
of women turn to the Internet if they have a private body question.

Source: Health.com poll

Loud, Louder, Loudest

How noisy is your everyday world? Here's how some sounds stack up*:

INJURY RANGE:	**165**	shot-gun blast
	140	jet taking off
	120	ambulance siren
RISK RANGE:	**110**	rock concert
	100	music from an iPod
	95	motorcycle
	85	heavy city traffic
SAFE RANGE:	**70**	washing machine
	60	normal conversation
	45	the humming of a refrigerator
	30	a quiet room, like a library

* In decibels

Q. I look exactly like a relative who died young. Does that mean I'll die young too?

Relax, you're not going to die any time soon—at least not because of how you look. You might share the same genes for appearance—the ones that gave you similar hair or eye color, facial features, or height—but that doesn't mean you share the genes for whatever was responsible for the death of your relative: cancer, heart disease, diabetes, etc.

But how close is this relative? If she was really close (like an aunt or grandmother), it's a good idea to find out what she died from and be screened for it or its precursors. In fact, you should do this for all your close relatives, regardless of whether or not you look like them. That way, even if you do have the same condition, you're ahead of the game and can get treatment or make the proper adjustments in your lifestyle (losing weight, exercising, etc.) to help you beat it. After all, to be forewarned is to be forearmed!

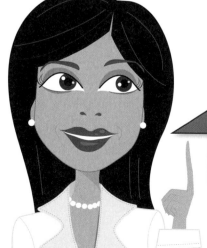

PSST, FROM DR. RAJ!
Using tech gadgets before bed can stimulate your brain and disrupt your sleep. So turn off the cell phone and laptop at least 20 minutes before bedtime and keep them out of the bedroom.

Q. My dentist says my old fillings can cause neurological problems and need to be replaced as soon as possible with porcelain ones. Is that for real?

While amalgam fillings (the old "silver" kind) do sometimes contain small amounts of mercury, the amounts that could possibly be released into your bloodstream are so minute there's almost no reason to be concerned. The American Dental Association still supports the use of amalgam as a safe, reliable way to treat tooth decay. And researchers have been unable to find any problems connected to the mercury in your fillings. So there's no health reason to replace them. Of course, if you grind your teeth and have fillings, you increase the chances you're releasing a little bit of mercury (from grinding away at the filling), so if you're really concerned you should ask your dentist about wearing a mouth guard at night.

Q. That's me! I grind my teeth, and I have fillings. Should I be checked for mercury poisoning?

You don't have to be checked, but if you're losing sleep over this issue, it's worth talking to your doctor about a blood-level mercury test, even if it's only to put your mind at ease. Or you can ask your dentist to remove them if that eases your mind. But the fact is, the small amounts of mercury in a filling aren't nearly enough to cause you any health problems.

NORMAL OR NOT:
Phantom buzzing in pocket from cell phones

Normal. Imagining that your phone is vibrating in your pocket doesn't mean you're crazy. It just means you need to unplug from your phone. Give it a rest every now and then.

Q. Are energy-efficient bulbs making people crazy?

Nope. This is one of those Internet rumors that has a germ of basis in fact. Compact fluorescent lights (CFLs) do contain mercury, which can cause neurological damage, especially if you eat it. But you're not eating these light bulbs (I hope)! As long as the bulb is intact, you're not exposed to mercury so there's no danger. Of course, you *do* need to be very careful if you break a CFL—air out the room, and don't touch the pieces of the bulb or any of the contents with your bare hands (just like with an old-school mercury thermometer). And when you change a CFL bulb, be sure to recycle it according to regulations in your area—you don't want to expose your trash collector to any mercury from broken bulbs.

Overall, CFLs actually reduce mercury emissions in the environment because they use less energy. Coal-burning power plants emit mercury, so less energy used means less mercury exposure over time.

· · · · · · ·

PLANTS
Can Detox Your Home!

Instead of heavy air fresheners, try nature's purifier: plants. Peace lilies remove toxins like acetone, benzene, alcohols, and ammonia from the air. To get rid of formaldehyde indoors, add a few bamboo palms and rubber plants. Also great: English ivy and Lady palm.

Q. Are plastic bottles really so bad?

It's looking that way. You've probably heard talk of BPA (or Bisphenol-A). It's a chemical used in the manufacture of many hard plastics such as food containers and baby bottles. When news spread of the potentially harmful effects of this chemical (including reproductive problems and even cancer), people began to worry, and companies began touting their BPA-free products like mad. But recently there has been evidence that some other chemicals in plastics might also have harmful health effects, and these chemicals are present even in BPA-free bottles and containers.

How do these chemicals get into our bodies? Heating plastic (like in the microwave) increases the potential for the plastic to release toxins into your food or drink. Chemicals can be released from plastic packing material, even the bags that seal microwave meals.

Plastic utensils might also release chemicals if they get hot.

My advice? Until we know more, use plastic in moderation. When it's convenient, opt for glass or ceramic over plastic, and avoid heating plastic in the microwave. Drinking from a plastic bottle once in a while is fine, but for daily use I'd use a glass or stainless steel bottle.

5 billion
The number of texts Americans send a day.

Source: Health.com poll

• • • • • • •

Q. I think my fingertips are going numb from always being on my BlackBerry. Should I be worried?

Step away from the Crackberry! Too much texting can cause a host of problems: back pain from poor posture; elbow or wrist pain from supporting the weight of the phone and the position of your arm when you talk or type; and tendonitis or even arthritis from repeated pressure on your fingertips.

Consider the numbness a warning sign to cut back on your chatting, texting, and typing or you could have serious problems down the road. If it persists or you start developing pain or numbness in your hands or arms, see your doctor to make sure you don't have a neurological problem.

• • • • • • •

Q. Won't the iPad really mess up your neck, since it's flat and you're looking straight down at it?

It could. Maintaining good posture is always important when using a computer. Laptops and iPads should not be used on your lap for long periods because they can cause neck and back strain. So just as the best way to use a laptop is on a desk with the screen at eye level and the keyboard easily reachable, the best place for an iPad, Kindle, or other screen device is propped or held up at or just below eye level. It may not sound very cool, but consider getting a stand for long-term use to prevent neck and back aches.

INDEX

INDEX

INDEX

Oxmoor House

VP, Publishing Director: Jim Childs
Editorial Director: Susan Payne Dobbs
Brand Manager: Fonda Hitchcock
Managing Editor: Laurie S. Herr

What the Yuck?!

Editor: Katherine Cobbs
Project Editor: Emily Chappell
Production Manager: Greg Amason

Contributors

Art Director/Illustrator: Ben Margherita
Compositor: Teresa Cole
Reporter: Kimberly Holland
Factchecker: Julie Gillis
Copy Editor: Dolores Hydock
Medical Reviewers: Dr. C. Glenn Cobbs, MD, and Dr. Mark Ricketts, MD
Proofreader: Norma Buttersworth McKittrick
Indexer: Mary Pelletier-Hunyadi

To order additional publications, call
1-800-765-6400 or 1-800-491-0551.

For more books to enrich your life, visit **oxmoorhouse.com**

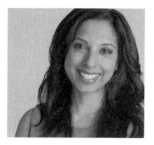

ROSHINI RAJAPASKA, MD

is board certified in Gastroenterology and Internal Medicine, with a medical degree from New York University School of Medicine and an undergraduate degree from Harvard College. Dr. Raj is an attending physician at NYU Langone Medical Center/Tisch Hospital in New York City, where she was the first female gastroenterologist to join the faculty.

She also serves as an Assistant Professor of Medicine, and has a special interest in women's health and cancer screening. She has published several research articles on colon cancer screening.

Dr. Raj has discussed a wide variety of health topics on NBC's *TODAY* show, ABC's *Good Morning America* and *World News Tonight*, CNN's *American Morning*, *Nancy Grace*, and *Larry King Live*, Discovery *Health*, the *Tyra Show*, *The Dr. Oz Show*, and many other national programs.

She is currently a *TODAY* show medical contributor and Medical Editor of *Health* magazine.

She has been quoted in *The New York Times*, *The Wall Street Journal*, *Cosmopolitan*, *Men's Health*, *Women's Health*, *Fitness*, and other publications on the state of health-care issues and health news of the day.

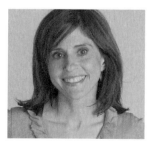

LISA LOMBARDI

is the Executive Editor of *Health* magazine and a blogger at Health.com. A Yale graduate, she has written extensively about health and lifestyle topics for leading publications and websites including *Glamour*, *The New York Times*, *Marie Claire*, *Maxim*, *Redbook*, *Child*, msn.com, and *Cosmopolitan*. She was the founding Editor-in-Chief of the teen magazine *Twist*, and has appeared as a guest expert on national TV and radio shows. She lives in the New York City area with her husband and two young sons.